*A Natural Approach*

# Arthritis

**Macrobiotic Health Education Series**

*A Natural Approach*

# Arthritis

*by* Michio Kushi

*edited by* Charles Millman

*foreword by* David Dodson, M.D.

**Japan Publications, Inc.**
Tokyo · New York

MACROBIOTIC HEALTH EDUCATION SERIES

*Note to the reader:* Those with health problems are advised to seek the guidance of a qualified medical, or psychological professional in addition to that of a qualified macrobiotic counselor before implementing any of the dietary and other approaches presented in this book. It is essential that any reader who has any reason to suspect serious illness in themselves or their family members seek appropriate medical, nutritional, or psychological advice promptly. Neither this or any other health related book should be used as a substitute for qualified care or treatment.

Published by JAPAN PUBLICATIONS, INC., Tokyo & New York

*Distributors:*
UNITED STATES: *Kodansha International/USA, Ltd., through Harper & Row, Publishers, Inc., 599 Lexington Avenue, Suite 2300, New York, N. Y. 10022.* SOUTH AMERICA: *Harper & Row, Publishers, Inc., International Department.* CANADA: *Fitzhenry & Whiteside Ltd., 195 Allstate Parkway, Markham, Ontario, L3R 4T8.* MEXICO AND CENTRAL AMERICA: *HARLA S. A. de C. V., Apartado 30–546, Mexico 4, D. F.* BRITISH ISLES: *Premier Book Marketing Ltd., 1 Gower Street, London WC1E 6HA.* EUROPEAN CONTINENT: *European Book Service PBD, Strijkviertel 63, 3454 PK De Meern, The Netherlands.* AUSTRALIA AND NEW ZEALAND: *Bookwise International, 54 Crittenden Road, Findon, South Australia 5007.* THE FAR EAST AND JAPAN: *Japan Publications Trading Co., Ltd., 1–2–1, Sarugaku-cho, Chiyoda-ku, Tokyo 101.*

First edition: November 1988

*LCCC No. 88–081559*
*ISBN 0–87040–676–0*

Printed in U.S.A.

# Foreword

Just over one-hundred years ago, the notion that invisible, micro-
scopic "germs" caused disease would have been considered completely
crackpot. By the 1880s though, brilliant men such as Lister, Pasteur,
and Koch had conclusively demonstrated that microbes do indeed
cause numerous conditions including tuberculosis, malaria, and even
leprosy. Today many people doubt the importance of diet and health,
particularly doctors! In fact, the Arthritis Foundation recently
distributed a pamphlet which stated, "The truth about diet and
arthritis may surprise you. It is simply this: There is NO special diet
for arthritis. No specific food has anything to do with causing it.
And no specific diet will cure it."

Even the Arthritis Foundation no longer believes this nonsense,
but nevertheless many doctors still believe that diet plays only a
minor role, if any at all, in arthritis, or in most other conditions for
that matter. Let us briefly examine why I referred to the above quote
as nonsense.

First of all, arthritis means inflammation of joints. Medicine now
recognizes about one hundred different types of arthritis: rheumatoid
arthritis, gout, and post-traumatic arthritis are just three examples.
No matter what type of arthrtis you have though, the more you
weigh, the more your joints are likely to hurt. If you have a sore knee
or ankle, you surely will not want to carry a fifty-pound sack of flour
around. Unfortunately, overweight arthritics carry around pounds
they cannot get rid of as easily as setting down a a sack of flour.
Macrobiotics is definitely the ultimate weight-loss diet, and solving
any weight problem will automatically make the overweight arthritic
more comfortable.

There are at least two other mechanisms by which a macrobiotic
diet can help arthritis sufferers. The first deals with a group of substances known as *autocoids*, or locally acting hormones. The best
known autocoids are the *prostaglandins*. There are numerous different
types of prostaglandins produced throughout the body which regulate
inflammation and other vital functions. The prostaglandins ultimately derive from the food we eat and therefore, by changing the
kinds of food we eat, we also change the prostaglandins and other
autocoids in our bodies. This has been shown to have a beneficial
effect on arthritis as reported in Britain's prestigious medical journal
*The Lancet*, on January 24, 1985. More specifically, it appears that

animal fats are converted into the types of prostaglandins that increase inflammation.

Finally, there is the issue of food allergy. Food allergy is an extremely confusing issue in medicine, so confusing in fact, that many doctors do not believe it exists. This is principally because the symptoms of food allergy can occur up to three weeks after eating the offending food and because many, if not most patients, are allergic to not just one but to several foods. Thus, if Mary has arthritis caused by allergy to eggs, milk, and tomatoes, and she eliminates eggs and milk but not tomatoes, she may fail to get better and may mistakenly believe that she is not allergic to milk and eggs. Furthermore, if Mary were careful not to consume any eggs, milk, or tomatoes for two weeks and failed to get better, she might conclude erroneously—though not unreasonably—that she was not allergic to these foods. The problem is, as mentioned above, that allergic symptoms may occur up to three weeks after eating the allergen, or allergy causing substance.

It has now been clearly demonstrated that several types of arthritis are related to food allergy. Interestingly, the first reliable report in the medical literature was a report which appeared in the *Annals of Allergy* in 1969. The author of the article, Dr. Stephan Epstein, had carefully documented the fact that his own case of palindromic rheumatism was caused by allergy to peppermint and to nitrites, a common food additive. It is curious that this fascinating and thorough report failed to convince more doctors of the importance of food allergy, particularly considering that the author and patient was himself a physician.

The macrobiotic diet avoids the common food allergens: milk, eggs, and sugar are the "big three." As illustrated by Dr. Epstein, food additives can be the allergen in some cases, and therefore the macrobiotic principle of using only the best quality, organic food is also important for those who suffer from arthritis and other conditions that may be caused by food allergy. A warning though: you may find you are allergic to some good macrobiotic foods. For example, fish and strawberries, either of which can be consumed occasionally by most macrobiotic people, are two fairly common food allergens.

I hope this brief discussion serves to dispell the old idea most doctors were taught in medical school that diet has nothing to do with arthritis. Diet has much to do with arthritis and perhaps most other diseases as well. As a physician and a nutritionist, I see the connection in terms of allergies, autocoids, and so on. To the macrobiotic teacher, the connection may be expressed in terms of the traditional Oriental view. To look at the subject both ways is to see the Yin and the Yang, to see the big picture. It is only by looking at the big picture that we can hope to successfully deal with big problems, such as the problem of arthritis.

David Dodson, M.D.
Boston, Massachusetts

# Introduction

Athritits represents one part of the worldwide epidemic of degenerative diseases that challenges humanity in the latter part of the twentieth century. Cancer, heart disease, AIDS, mental illness, and other degenerative sicknesses are not confined by national borderlines. They have spread to every corner of our planet without passports or visas.

Although the number of people in the United States with arthritis is officially estimated at 37 million, the actual number is much higher when we include those with undiagnosed arthritis, or add those with the condition referred to as *pre-arthritis*, or the unnatural stiffening of the joints that often begins in childhood. For many people today, especially senior citizens, the pain of arthritis is a constant companion. As a result, the idea has become prevalent that arthritis is a natural part of the aging process. Although this concept is generally accepted in modern society, it deserves to be thoroughly questioned, as does the notion that the process of aging is one in which a multitude of other chronic conditions, such as cancer, heart disease, Alzheimer's disease, and others, are the inevitable result.

In macrobiotics we take the view that these and other degenerative conditions are not natural or normal, but occur because we have forgotten how to eat and live in harmony with the environment. The macrobiotic way of life is fundamental in restoring harmony with nature, so that each stage in life—from infancy to old age—can be one of natural health, productive activity, and joyous fulfillment.

Increasingly, the prevention of chronic illness has become a leading social issue, as the crisis of AIDS and immune deficiencies has shown. As we move toward the next century, an increasing percentage of the population of the United States and other modern nations will become older, especially as the postwar baby-boom generation reaches middle age. Therefore, the choices made now, in terms of diet, lifestyle, and our overall approach to health and sickness, could soon determine the quality of life for society as a whole.

The choices we face are becoming clear: we can continue on the present path without changing our way of life, and risk developing cancer, heart disease, arthritis, or some other life-threatening or disabling condition; or we can take positive action now to improve our daily life—and especially our daily diet—in order to prevent these conditions and enjoy health and productivity throughout life.

The road we choose could determine the quality of life not just for individuals in the immediate future, but for generations to come.

This book, as well as the other titles in the *Macrobiotic Health Education Series*, has been written in order to provide an alternative to the decline of modern civilization through degenerative disease. The dietary recommendations of macrobiotics are now being echoed in preventive guidelines for cancer, heart disease, and other degenerative disorders issued by leading public health agencies throughout the world. Moreover, hundreds of thousands of people—from Tokyo to Texas, and from Utah to Yugoslavia—have embraced its principles. Many have experienced the recovery of health, including the improvement of arthritis and other crippling diseases, as a result.

As you will discover, macrobiotics offers more than just a naturally balanced diet. The principles explained in this book offer a new view of human life and health, a view that is in accord with thousands of years of traditional understanding found in both East and West. The application of these universal principles can open the door to a new era in our understanding of health and sickness, and pave the way toward the development of a medicine for all of humanity.

I would like to thank everyone who contributed to the completion of this book. I thank our friend and associate, Edward Esko, for coordinating the compilation and editing of the materials, and for adding insights based on many years of study and practice of the macrobiotic way of life. I also thank our associate, Charles Millman, for researching much of the information on arthritis and for applying macrobiotic principles to understanding the nature of this disorder.

I thank David Dodson, M.D., for contributing a foreword, together with our friends who contributed their personal recovery stories. I also thank Christian Gautier for his artwork and illustrations, as well as our associate, Phillip Jannetta, and the Japan Publications staff in Tokyo for editing and proofreading the text. I express appreciation to Aveline Kushi and Wendy Esko for compiling the companion cookbook in the *Macrobiotic Food and Cooking Series*, and thank Mr. Iwao Yoshizaki and Mr. Yoshiro Fujiwara, president and New York representative of Japan Publications, for their continuing support of macrobiotic publishing projects.

Michio Kushi
Brookline, Massachusetts
April, 1988

# Contents

# 1. The Mystery of Arthritis

Today, we are faced with a health problem that seems a mystery. It is not a new problem. For thousands of years humanity has attempted to understand it. Yet, despite the efforts of the finest minds, past and present, the help of today's advanced technology, and the expenditure of hundreds of millions of dollars for research, the riddle remains unsolved. As a consequence, each of us is likely to personally experience this problem to some degree in our lifetime. Because we cannot solve it, we cannot avoid it. This is the mystery of arthritis.

Currently there are about 37 million people in the United States who have been officially diagnosed with arthritis. If we add to this the number of people who suffer from arthritis and have not yet been medically diagnosed, the new figure would be closer to 70 million. This represents nearly one-third of the population of the United States. And even this does not reveal the full extent of arthritis. As each of us grows older, our chances of getting arthritis increase. In fact, it is believed that almost everyone over the age sixty has arthritic changes in their joints. Arthritis is a health issue that we cannot escape.

The purpose of this book is to reveal why arthritis has become part of our life pattern. In order to accomplish this, we must begin by finding the cause or origin. This is the key point because if we can understand the true cause of arthritis, we can then take the proper corrective measures to change or avoid it. To begin our search for a solution, we can examine what is presently known about arthritis, its suspected causes, the kinds of treatments used and their effectiveness, and how this degenerative disease changes us individually and collectively.

The word *arthritis* is derived from the Greek language. *Arth* means "joint," and *itis* means "inflammation." According to this definition, arthritis is an inflammation of one or more of the many joints in the body. At the time this definition was coined that may actually have been the dominant type of arthritis. Today however, with modern methods of diagnosis, the definition of arthritis takes into account much more than just an inflammation of the joints. It includes other types of joint and connective-tissue problems, plus a large number of additional bodily symptoms that can accompany arthritis.

Officially, arthritis is one disease that comes under the general heading of *rheumatic diseases*. *Rheumatism* is a Greek word derived from *rheumatisomos*, or the mucus which was believed to flow from the brain to the joints and other portions of the body, producing pain of varying degrees. Rheumatic diseases is a common term that covers pain and stiffness in some portion of the musculoskeletal system. This includes our joints and connective tissue. The general focus of this book is on arthritis, joint problems and accompanying symptoms, and specifically the major types of arthritis.

Arthritis is thought to be one of the oldest diseases afflicting human beings. Our ancestors, Ape man of two million years ago, suffered from chronic arthritis of the spine, as did our closer relatives, Java and Lansing man. X-ray examination of Egyptian mummies have revealed arthritis. Ramses II, who ruled Egypt from 1304 B.C. to 1225 B.C., suffered from arthritis. Hippocrates, the ancient Greek healer and father of moden medicine, knew about and treated arthritis. During the Roman Empire an extensive system of elaborate baths were built in order to ease the aches and pains of arthritis.

Some of the most famous and familiar historical figures did not escape arthritis. These include: Christopher Columbus, Cardinal Richelieu, Mary Queen of Scots, President James Madison, Horace the Poet, Julius Caesar, Augustus Caesar, Pope Pius II, Leonardo DaVinci, Michaelangelo, Benjamin Franklin, and Martin Luther. Arthritis is a most democratic disease. It strikes the poet and the politician, the writer and the thinker, the actor and actress, and even the king and queen.

An amazing variety of treatments have been employed to ease the pain and suffering of arthritis. Acupuncture was used in China, certain African tribes used tattooing, and the Hindus of 1200 B.C. used a variety of methods such as liniments, leeches and bleeding. Hippocrates recommended draining swollen joints plus a dietary regimen that restricted wine and called for occasional purging. The Romans used herbal remedies, wine, wool fat, hot baths, fennel, flax seed, vinegar, limes, and other food items. Galen, a noted Roman physician, even prescribed a sharp cheese and pork application to the troubled joint. Arabs cauterized with hot irons. The Tibetans, Malayans, and Japanese all had their unique treatments. In fact, it seems that every major culture has tried an astonishing variety of remedies for arthritis.

From these diverse methods of treatment we can discern basic strategies underlying their use. First is the attempt to rid the body of excess through such regimens as purging with laxatives, vomiting, and dietary restrictions. The common thinking behind these methods was that arthritis is a form of bodily exess that could be eliminated. Once removed, the body would return to a normal condition. The reason for this strategy can be easily understood if one has ever seen a full, swollen, hot joint. The second general approach included specific treatments of the troubled area in the attempt to relieve the intense pain. The success of these treatments is not well documented. If one or any of them had been truly effective, they would probably be in use today. Of all of these, the two that remain with us are the idea of a dietary regimen and acupuncture.

Modern methods of treatment include a huge assortment of medications, as well as physical therapy and exercise. When these measures cannot produce a favorable result, then surgery is used. Although these methods can sometimes provide temporary relief, they are not able to fundamentally change the course of arthritis.

There are about 37 million officially diagnosed cases of arthritis in the United States today. A breakdown of the major types is given below.

| Type of Arthritis | Number of Cases | Incidence |
| --- | --- | --- |
| Gout | 1 million | 80% to 90% men |
| Rheumatoid Arthritis | 7 million | 75% women |
| Lupus and Arthritis | ¼ million | 8 to 10 times more women than men |
| Ankylosing Spondylitis | 2.5 million | Mostly men |
| Osteoarthritis | 16 million | Everyone over age 60 |

In addition, over 100 types of arthritis have been identified, and these can be divided into two large categories according to their basic effects on the joints and body as a whole. One category includes *inflammatory* kinds of arthritis. This group is distinguished by the symptoms of bodily or joint inflammation. Examples include rheumatoid arthritis, *tenosynovitis, lupus erythematous, polymyositis, dermatomyositis, psoriatic arthritis,* and many others. The other category is *noninflammatory*. This designation means that for the most part, these types of arthritis are not characterized by inflammation. Among these are *primary osteoarthritis* and *isolated osteoarthritis, traumatic arthritis, pseudogout, neuroarthropathy, enthesopathy,* and *tendonitis*. However, this division is not without exceptions. At times, there can be inflammation in one of the noninflammatory types. This greatly contributes to the difficulty in making a clear diagnosis.

Arthritis can strike at any time in life. *Juvenile arthritis* strikes over 150,000 people under the age of sixteen. In fact, there are even recorded cases of arthritis among babies. As we age, the variety and incidence of arthritis increases. And in old age, arthritis becomes a constant companion. As a result, we have come to associate the debilitating effects of arthritis with aging. This is most distressing and sad. At a time when individuals should be enjoying the fruits of their life, they often experience pain, deformity, and a restriction of movement.

The prevalence of arthritis exacts a heavy toll on society. Millions upon millions of people cannot routinely perform the normal functions of daily life. And in severe cases, many cannot work and support themselves. What is the toll of arthritis? One way to assess the multiple effects of arthritis is to examine its economic impact.

Table 1   Some Economic Costs of Arthritis

| | |
|---|---|
| *Direct Costs of Medical Care, Annual* | |
| Hospitalization | $1,431,000,000 |
| Physical visits | 1,238,000,000 |
| Services from other health professionals | 322,000,000 |
| Drugs | 798,000,000 |
| Nursing home care | 679,000,000 |
| Unproven remedies | 1,758,000,000 |
| Total, direct | $6,226,000,000 |
| *Indirect Costs of Medical Care, Annual* | |
| Lost wages | $6,046,000,000 |
| Lost homemaker services | 661,000,000 |
| Lost wages and homemaker services for institutionalized people | 239,000,000 |
| Earning lost due to early death | 97,000,000 |
| Total, indirect | $7,043,000,000 |
| Total Annual Economic Costs | $13,269,000,000 |

These figures have been extrapolated for 1982 from National Center for Health Statistics' *Health Interview Survey, Nursing Home Survey* and *Hospital Discharge Survey*, 1975.

Thirteen billion dollars in annual expenditures is the figure that jumps from the page. And since arthritis is increasing by about one million new cases a year, this figure is constantly rising.

The category of direct costs refers to the actual costs spent for arthritis, such as doctor's visits, hospitalization, drugs, medical tests, and others. The bottom half of the chart lists indirect costs. In many cases, someone with arthritis cannot work on a regular basis because of pain, and as a result, valuable services are lost. If the condition is severe, an individual may be institutionalized. These indirect costs do not include lost taxes, disability payments, and other expenses that would substantially increase the annual cost of arthritis. These figures show that huge economic resources are being channeled into this disease.

Numbers, no matter how large and how spectacular, do not reveal the personal side of arthritis. What does arthritis mean for individuals? How does it effect their quality of life and personal relationships?

Waking up in the morning and immediately facing pain is not a prospect anyone would relish. But for the arthritis patient, this can be a daily part of life. The simplest acts, such as getting out of bed in the morning and walking to the bathroom and brushing our teeth, which we all take for granted, can be painful acts of courage and endurance. Going through a day with chronic or intermittent pain is physically, mentally, and emotionally draining. Pain can make it difficult for someone to focus on tasks that must be performed. Arthritis can color someone's life and all of its parts.

Family relationships can become strained because of arthritis. If the man or woman of the house suffers from arthritis, the other partner may be called upon for extra patience, work, and devotion. If a child has arthritis, it creates a constant source of worry for the parents, And for the child, he or she could be deprived of normal participation in the school and play activities that are important for full development.

More intimate relationships may also change. The capacity for spontaneous initiation and response is altered by physical disability and pain. As a result, this situation requires special understanding and effort to avoid possible conflict.

The talent, abilities, and potential of a significant number of people are diminished because of arthritis. Society's most important resource is the health, strength, and vitality of its people. With these qualities intact, almost any difficulty can be overcome. When they are reduced because of sickness, that society is greatly weakened.

# 2. Major Types of Arthritis ━━━━━

In all types of arthritis, the joint is the common, basic problem. This makes a clear understanding of joints, their anatomy and functioning, a prerequisite to understanding the nature of arthritis. In the following diagram we can see the structure of a normal joint.

**Fig. 1   A Normal Joint**

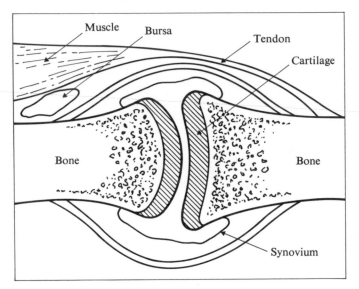

When a joint is normal and healthy, it permits a wide range of motions depending on its location in the body.

A joint is the place where two bones meet. There are many joints in the body. The spine is a long alignment of bones and joints stretching vertically. The hips, knees, ankles, and feet all contain joints, as do the shoulders, elbows, wrists, and hands. Where these bones meet, nature has provided a cushion. A disc made of more dense material forms a pad between spinal vertebrae. Other joints, such as the knees and elbows, have a more fluid cushion consisting of a *synovial membrane* within which *synovial fluid* lubricates the joint.

As the joint moves, the action of the two bones is further padded by cartilage covering each end of the bones. Movement of the joints causes a flushing action of the fluid that brings in fresh fluid and nutrients. Outside the joint lie supporting structures: the muscles, tendons, and ligaments that firmly anchor the joint in place during movement. The *bursa* is a small sac that cushions joint action.

The major function of the joint is to provide the capacity for general movement of the body. If our bodies were one solid piece, we could not bend, and movement would be nearly impossible. Joints provide us with freedom of movement in life; their health determines how much of this freedom we can enjoy. There is no action or movement that we perform in our daily life that does not depend upon our joints. In this sense, movement, as designed by nature, helps keep our joints healthy rather than wearing them out.

In addition to general movement, joints have particularized and refined movements. Some joints operate as a ball and socket, while others permit a rotational type of movement, and some act like a hinge. Of all the joints in the body, those of the hands give us the ability of very refined movement, such as playing the guitar or piano, painting, and writing.

All joints have the general capacity to bear and transfer weight. The larger joints of the lower spine, hips, and knees are designed to bear very large amounts of weight. In addition to supporting our bodily bulk, anything that we pick up and carry strongly presses down on these joints. This contrasts with the smaller joints of the upper part and periphery of the body, especially the hands and elbows. Their design is suited more for refined movement. Although they are capable of carrying and transferring weight, this ability is limited in comparison to the larger, lower-body joints.

What can go wrong with the joints? Just about everything you can think of and more. Every part of the joint can have problems: the cartilage, the synovial membrane, the fluid, the tendons, the bursae, and the ligaments are all subject to arthritis. Because nature has packed so much into such a small space, there can be a huge variety of problems.

Our ability to move, to do, to accomplish in life depends upon the health of our joints. The impression we give to others, how we present ourselves, and how we move become our signature by which other people identify us. The condition of our joints forms part of this basic nature and personality. When we have a joint problem, the perception that others have of us is changed. Seeing someone who is bent over, twisted, or who walks with a shuffle or limp creates a vivid image of infirmity and weakness. On the other hand, when our joints are healthy we stand erect and move smoothly, thus projecting an impression of youth, vitality, and strength.

In addition to basic joint problems, there can be a large number of accompanying symptoms, depending on which type of arthritis strikes. These can range from almost total body involvement, such as in lupus, to very few accompanying symptoms as in osteoarthritis. Each of these adds to the difficulty of diagnosis and also the effectiveness of treatment.

With this background we can now look at the major types of arthritis and see their specific symptomatic patterns.

## Rheumatoid Arthritis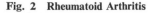

Sir Alfred Baring Garrod, a British M.D., was the originator of the name *rheumatoid arthritis*. He selected the word "rheumatoid" to describe this type of arthritis because of the similarity of its symptoms to rheumatic fever, especially in the early stages. Rheumatoid arthritis is primarily an inflammation of the joint areas of the body, specifically the synovial membrane which wraps around the joint. Together with expansion of the membrane, the volume of joint fluid also increases.

Fig. 2  Rheumatoid Arthritis

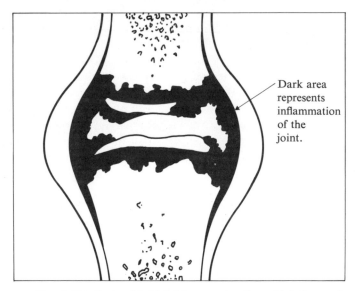

Dark area represents inflammation of the joint.

In rheumatoid arthritis, the troubled joint becomes swollen with inflammation of the synovial membrane.

In rheumatoid arthritis, cells in the synovial membrane divide and grow as inflammatory cells come into the joint from other parts of the body. As a result, the joint becomes swollen and stiff. Increased blood flow makes the joint warm. Enzymes are released from cells into the joint space and add to the pain and irritation. The initial symptoms are usually pain when moving the joint or pain upon arising. If this process is allowed to continue unchecked, the cartilage and bone are eroded, leading to joint deformation and eventual rigidity.

The knuckles and wrists are almost always involved in rheumatoid arthritis. The knee and the joint of the ball of the foot are the next most frequent areas of involvement. It is possible for almost any joint to be afflicted.

Rheumatoid arthritis is not a localized disease. The whole body is affected. Accompanying symptoms can include low fever, fatigue, and loss of appetite and weight. Anemia in varying degrees can be present, especially in severe cases. The lung can be involved with possible *pleurisy*, an inflammation of the membrane that lines the chest and covers the lungs. The spleen can be enlarged with irregular white blood cell production. Possible *tachycardia*, or rapid heart action, can occur. Cold, moist, tingling hands and feet, and excessive sweating are also possible. Lumps under the skin, called *rheumatoid nodules*, can grow to the size of a pea or mothball, especially in the elbow area.

For the majority of rheumatoid arthritis patients, the disease is chronic. However, there are two other patterns to be considered. The first is when a person experiences a brief bout of rheumatoid arthritis, which then mysteriously recedes and does not come back. This is called *monocyclic*. The second is a cycle of pain and illness followed by a period when the person feels normal before the next bout of pain returns. This is called *polycyclic*.

Rheumatoid arthritis stikes roughly two to three females for every male. About 75 percent of the cases occur in women. The age of onset peaks between thirty-six and forty-five years of age.

In order to confirm a diagnosis of rheumatoid arthritis, a variety of medical tests can be used. In 80 percent of all cases, the *rheumatoid factor* or *latex* proves positive. This test searches for an antibody to certain body proteins. Also, a sedimentation test is administered. This shows the rate at which the heavier elements of the blood settle. A high sed rate is an indication of a serious condition. Finally, X-rays determine the damage to bone and cartilage.

The major treatment used for rheumatoid arthritis is aspirin. It can be used either as an *analgesic*, which means "pain reliever," or as an *anti-inflammatory agent*. For aspirin to work, a blood level of 18 to 25 milligrams percent is required. For this blood level to be maintained, 12 to 25 five-grain aspirin tablets must be taken daily. Although aspirin is the drug used most in treating rheumatoid arthritis, other medications may also be administered. A physician can select which drug to use based on the severity of the disease and the patient's response to medication. The ability of a patient to tolerate whatever drug is given must be taken into careful consideration and closely monitored because these drugs are taken over an extended period of time and in larger doses if the arthritis is particularly severe.

In addition to drugs, physical therapy is important to keep joints mobile. Such treatments as heat packs, cold packs, warm baths, and *diathermy* (high frequency electrical heat treatment) are also used.

A program of self-exercise can be prescribed. These exercises are performed when the patient is capable of moving a damaged joint or joints. Exercise aids circulation and helps keep joints mobile.

Rest is also important when physical movement is restricted by pain. Daily, constant pain is draining and fatiguing, and usually demands extra rest.

## Lupus

Lupus is a disease of multiple symptoms, one of which can be arthritis. The complete name for this disease is *systemic lupus erythematosus*. But either the term "lupus" or the initials "SLE" are used to designate it. Lupus itself is a connective tissue disease. The autoimmune system, which normally protects the body, begins to destroy healthy tissue. The reason this happens is not known.

The symptoms of lupus can involve a large portion of the body. A butterfly rash over the bridge of the nose and cheeks can arise. *Raynaud's phenomenon*, a change in the color of the hands, can take place. There can be a rapid loss of large amounts of scalp hair. The skin is usually reactive to direct sunlight. There can be ulcers in the mouth. *Proteinuria*, the loss of excessive amounts of protein in the urine, can happen. *Pleuritis* can strike with a thickening and inflammation of the pleural lining. *Pericarditis*, or the inflammation of the heart area, can also occur. In addition, inflammation of the *peritoneum*, the membrane around the abdominal cavity, can take place.

One half of lupus patients have *nephritis*, the collection inside the kidneys of immune complements from autoantibodies. Blood cell counts are also affected. The red blood cells can be depressed, leading to anemia. White blood cells can also be lowered.

In addition to these possible symptoms of lupus, there can be arthritis. The arthritis of lupus strikes the synovial membrane of the joint. This is similar to rheumatoid arthritis, although the symptoms differ in degree. The joints do not usually swell in cases of lupus and the condition is not as severe as in rheumatoid arthritis. There is tenderness and pain on motion. The joints affected by lupus are the same as rheumatoid arthritis. The wrists and knuckles, especially the middle finger, and the knees in the lower part of the body are most often afflicted. The spine is usually not involved.

A striking factor of lupus incidence is that over 90 percent of lupus cases occur in women in their childbearing years. As a result, there is an increased chance of miscarriage, especially in the early part of pregnancy. After delivery, there can be a worsening of symptoms.

Tests used to diagnose lupus may include a blood count, urine analysis, X-rays, an electrocardiogram or echocardiogram. These tests are in addition to a basic physical examination.

The drugs used to treat lupus depend on the severity of the case. Cortisone and immunosuppressives are used in serious cases. Other drugs used are the anti-inflammatory agents—aspirin and hydro-oxychloroquine.

## Osteoarthritis

Osteoarthritis is like a long, slow decay that eats away at the cartilage of the joints. Over a period of time the cartilage becomes pitted and frayed, losing its smooth surface and ability to pad the movement of the two bones. As this erosion increases, the cartilage can be totally worn away and the exposed ends of the bones can rub against each other. The exposed bony ends thicken and form bony growths that cement the bones together.

This sort of arthritis is distinguished from other types by several factors. There is no or little inflammation in osteoarthritis. Its onset is slow and insidious, rather than the more intense cyclic nature of other varieties of arthritis. And there are generally no accompanying symptoms. In the past this type of arthritis was assumed to be part of the aging process. Today however, this theory is being re-examined and newer theories are surfacing that question this assumption.

Part of the reason that osteoarthritis was thought to be part of the aging process is the extent of its prevalence as one grows older. By age forty, 90 percent of all persons have degenerative changes in their weight-bearing joints. And by age sixty, practically no one is exempt. Although these changes take place, many people do not experience strong enough symptoms to register an official complaint.

The primary target of osteoarthritis seems to be the weight-bearing

## Fig. 3   Osteoarthritis

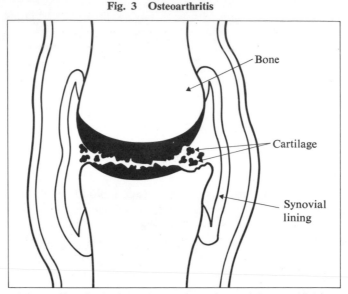

Bone

Cartilage

Synovial
lining

Erosion of the cartilage in the joints is a common feature of osteoarthritis.

joints. The hips, knees, feet, and spine are most often struck. Bony growths can appear in the neck or the lower back along the spine. The spinal vertebrae narrow and the disc which is a cushion between them is diminished. In the upper part of the body, the ends of the fingers are most often affected. A bony enlargement at the fingertip joint is referred to as *Heberden's nodes*. There can also be a bony enlargement on the second joint of the fingers, called *Bouchard's nodes*. The fingers can become bent, bony, and stiff.

A diagnosis of osteoarthritis is usually made by X-rays that show the space between the two bones of the joint narrowing and eventually coming together. Also, the appearance of nodes on the fingertip joints and the patient's description of the pain are used. In general, blood tests register normal in osteoarthritis.

Prescribed treatment of osteoarthritis is a program of exercise to increase the range of joint motion and flexibility. Aspirin in moderate doses is taken, and anti-inflammatory drugs are also recommended at times. To relieve the joint pain, hot and cold treatments can be used.

## Ankylosing Spondylitis

The arthritis of ankylosing spondylitis, or *AS*, occurs when inflammatory cells invade the area where a tendon or ligament attaches to the bone. After the initial inflammation, a bony ridge grows between the joints so that they become fused. This process takes place along the spine.

### Fig. 4 Normal Vertebrae

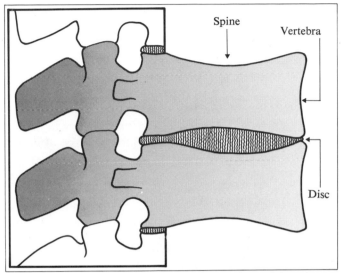

Normally the disc provides a cushion between the vertebrae of the spine.

### Fig. 5 Ankylosing Spondylitis

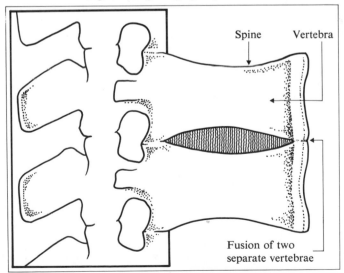

In ankylosing spondylitis, the disc area shrinks as the vertebrae contract and fuse.

Ankylosing spondylitis strikes the lower sacroiliac joints of the spine first. Then the disease gradually moves up the spine. The result of this is usally described by the terms "poker spine" or "bamboo spine." However, these terms are not entirely accurate because a poker is straight and bamboo grows straight. The effect of this disease on a human being is different. It does not make a person erect and rigid. Instead the spine becomes bent, looking as if someone is carrying a great burden and bent forward under the weight. The eyes are pointed to the ground, the chest region is collapsed, and the ability to take a full stride is diminished because the fused joints of the lower spine do not permit full natural extension of the hip region. This kind of posture is what we associate with older people, hunched over with shuffling gait, and using a cane to steady them as they move.

Ankylosing spondylitis is not a rapid or intense type of disease. The typical age of onset is between sixteen and thirty-five years old. Deterioration continues for a long period of time before being discovered. This type of arthritis primarily strikes men.

The accompanying symptoms of AS are minor compared to other forms of arthritis. Fatigue and weight loss can be part of it. With severe cases there is inflammation of the eye causing pain and redness. In some patients, the aortic valve of the heart is afflicted.

In diagnosing ankylosing spondylitis, a genetic factor has been discovered. The antigen *JLA B 26* has been found in over 80 percent of all AS cases. This serves for identification and is not a causative agent. In addition, X-rays are used to check for fusion of the spinal joints.

The primary treatment for AS is physical therapy and specific exercises to maintain mobility and joint flexibility. Aspirin is not effective in AS cases.

# Gout

Throughout history a galaxy of brilliant men have suffered from gout. Among them are Benjamin Franklin, Michaelangelo, Leonardo DaVinci, Milton, Sir Issac Newton, and Charles Darwin. They suffered from one of the most intensely painful types of arthritis. The progress of gout follows a pattern. First, there is an elevation of *uric acid* in the blood. Uric acid is normally produced by the body as part of the metabolic process, although amounts fluctuate. Stress, puberty in boys, and menopause in women increase uric-acid levels. If there is a continuous, excessive amount in the blood, uric acid changes to crystals that deposit in joints and other tissues. These crystals are composed of sodium urate. Each crystal deposit is called a *tophus*. Deposits in the joints result in the extreme, bulbous swelling of the joint, with inflammation. It is not only the joints that are afflicted, however. There can be tophi inside the kidneys that may form kidney stones.

The sudden onset of a gout attack causes an extraordinary amount of pain. Commonly, the first attack begins at night. The pattern of attacks follow a cycle. At first, there is an intense attack that can last a few days. This can be followed by a period of up to two weeks in which the individual is symptom free before another attack. This timing sequence can vary from person to person but the general pattern of attack and relief is the initial sequence. Later, if the disease worsens, the joint pain does not go away.

Gout is a disease of the lower extremities. Ninety percent of gouty patients experience acute attacks in the large toe sometime during the course of their disease. A special name, *podgra*, is given to this particular type of attack.

**Fig. 6    Gout**

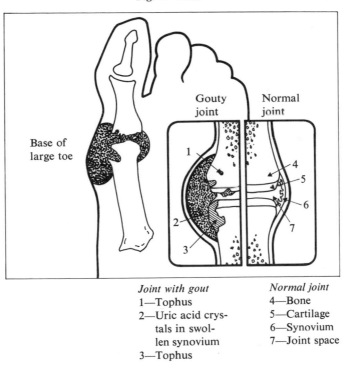

| Joint with gout | Normal joint |
|---|---|
| 1—Tophus | 4—Bone |
| 2—Uric acid crys- | 5—Cartilage |
| tals in swol- | 6—Synovium |
| len synovium | 7—Joint space |
| 3—Tophus | |

Gout usually occurs at the base of the large toe. Swollen, hot, and extremely painful, the joint space fills with needle-shaped crystals.

Other lower regions, such as the instep, ankles, heels, and knees, can be involved. In the upper part of the body, the wrists, fingers, and elbows can suffer gouty attacks. In some cases there are symptoms leading up to gout such as ankle sprains, sore heels, or twinges of pain in the large toe.

From our brief historical list, you may have noticed that the individuals are all males. This reflects the fact that the majority of gouty patients—80 to 90 percent—are men.

To confirm a diagnosis of gout, a test of the uric-acid levels in the blood will be administered, or a sample of joint fluid will be taken and examined for crystals.

Treatments for gout include a combination of diet and medication. This is because the dietary factor in gout has been recognized for quite some time. A diet high in meats, especially those which contain purines, is believed to bring on gout. That is because the metabolism cannot break down this excess. In addition to meat, overconsumption of alcohol is also linked to gout.

In relation to the dietary causes of gout, interesting epidemiological data appeared in the twentieth century. The incidence of gout greatly decreased during and just after the First and Second World Wars. During these periods there were food shortages and rationing, especially of richer food. Gout is also extremely rare among native people living in their original habitat. It is likely that their more natural, traditional lifestyle and diet are involved in their very low incidence of gout.

The first medication given for gout is usually *colchicine*. *Phenybutasone* and *indomethacin* are other anti-inflammatory agents that can be used. Sometimes corticosteroids are injected into the inflamed joint. Medicine to reduce the uric-acid levels between attacks is also given.

To avoid confusion, it should be mentioned that another form of arthritis, called *pseudogout*, also exists. Although it has similarities to gout, it is different in respect to the content of the crystals that develop in the joint. These are *pyrophosphate crystals*, and are composed more of calcium. This crystal buildup is slower in the body, making this condition more a problem for older persons. Seventy years is average for the first incidence. The knee is affected most often, with the wrists and ankles the next most involved joints. These attacks are not as clear cut and linger longer than gout.

# Modern Approaches to Arthritis ━━━━━━━━━

The approved treatments for arthritis today include medications, physical therapy, and exercise. When these measures are not sufficient, surgery is used as a last resort.

The use of medication is the current first line of treatment for arthritis. Drugs are used to relieve pain and to reduce inflammation. Because they have to be taken regularly to control symptoms, their use tends to become constant.

Aspirin is the number one medication used for arthritis. Of the 22 billion tablets of aspirin taken annually in this country, over half are consumed by arthritis sufferers. It is used to relieve pain and also to reduce inflammation. The inflammatory types of arthritis, such as rheumatoid arthritis and lupus, are treated primarily by aspirin.

Aspirin today is made from coal tar or petroleum from which its basic ingredient, *salicyclic acid*, is formed. An acetyl group of atoms is added to "tame" or reduce some of the toxic side effects of salicyclic acid. After blending and processing, this mixture is filtered and dried. Corn starch or talc are added as fillers. The aspirin to filler ratio can be 90 to 10 or 80 to 20 depending on the brand.

The current theory of how aspirin works is that it suppresses the the action of *prostaglandins*, which are naturally produced bodily substances that contain more than twenty hormones. Part of the function of prostaglandins is the reaction of pain and inflammation to bodily distress. Aspirin suppresses this normal reaction of prostaglandins and results in reduction of pain and inflammation.

In addition to aspirin, an assortment of other medications can be prescribed for particular types of arthritis. Depending on how severe a particular type of arthritis is, various drugs of different strengths can be prescribed.

A program of physical therapy is used to treat arthritis. Hot and cold packs, diathermy, baths, massage, the movement of the troubled joints by a therapist, and other techniques are attempted to relieve pain, to keep the joints flexible, and when possible, to increase their range of motion.

Arthritis patients are encouraged to follow, when possible, a program of self-exercise. The purpose is to keep joints mobile, which prevents stiffness, improves circulation, and increases the range of joint motion.

When medication, physical therapy, or self-exercise are not able to help, surgery is often used. Around 40,000 hip replacements are done annually in the United States. This number is increasing yearly. Stainless steel or vitalium plus plastic and polyethylene are the components used in the manufacture of artificial hip joints. In addition to the hip, which is the most commonly replaced joint, there are toe implants, finger, ankle, knee, knuckle, shoulder, and elbow joint replacements. Since these are less developed than hip replacements, their use has not yet become widespread.

Surgery does not mean that a person will no longer have arthritis. It means that because of arthritis, and the inability of other methods to control it, the diseased part must be cut out of the body. Even with the most troubled area removed and replaced, arthritis can still strike other parts of the body.

## Modern Theories About Arthritis ───────────

Cause is at the heart of the mystery of arthritis. Throughout history, some of the finest minds have tackled this issue and been unable to resolve it. Hippocrates, the father of modern medicine, Galen, a noted physician of Roman times, Benjamin Franklin, and many others have all offered possible causes. Yet none of these was effective in preventing or reversing arthritis. Today we have state-of-the-art, space-age technology to tackle this problem, including super computers to calculate and analyze results and powerful electron microscopes for seeing within the body. These and other technological marvels have yet to yield a definitive answer that would effectively treat this disease. As a result, there are many theories that attempt to explain the cause of arthritis.

One of the most persistent theories about the cause of arthritis is the *hereditary theory*, or the belief that people are born with the tendency to arthritis because of faulty genetic structure. This is suspected now in osteoarthritis. It is thought that inborn structural defects lead inevitably to this disease. As a result of research in this area, certain types of arthritis have been found to have genetic markers. It has been discovered that *HLA-DR4* can be correlated to rheumatoid arthritis. In ankylosing spondylitis, the genetic marker *HLA-B27* has been identified. This does not mean that every person with these markers will have arthritis. But since large numbers of people who have these markers also have arthritis, there is a proposed correlation between the two.

Another line of inquiry suggests that a triggering agent, such as a virus, is the cause. These triggering agents are waiting in our bodies for something that influences them to change and create arthritis.

Another school of thought sees various metabolic factors as possible causes of arthritis. *Metabolism* is the chemical and physical process by which food is built up into protoplasm and through which protoplasm is used and broken down into simpler substances of waste matter, as well as the release of energy for all vital processes from foodstuffs. These processes create metabolic factors that can be measured. For example, elevated levels of calcium have been found in rheumatoid arthritis patients. *Betaendomorphin*, a peptide in the brain, is deficient in some arthritis patients.

Microorganisms have also been implicated as a possible cause of arthritis. *Mycoplasmas* is one of the smallest phenomena in the body. It is neither a bacteria or a virus, but a class of petite organism that can reproduce without infecting a host. These tiny agents are thought to play a role in arthritis. *Substance P*, a short protein, is implicated in some arthritis cases. Generally, metabolic factors can be excessive or deficient. Their role in creating arthritis is not fully understood but is being studied.

The immune system is crucial to our general health and vitality. Our immune system helps the body neutralize foreign substances. Sometimes this system can begin to destroy healthy tissue, as in the case of lupus. What causes the immune system to malfunction in this manner is not yet understood.

There is a second area of arthritis inquiry that is relatively new and attracting very large interest. Perhaps it arose from the persistent yet basic question that people suffering from arthritis often ask, "Is it what I'm eating that is causing my problem?" In the past the idea of a diet and arthritis link was generally discounted. Except for gout, no food connection had been established in arthritis. This dismissal was premature because it took place without thorough and clear research and experimentation to test its possibility. However, this situation is changing.

In the publication *Arthritis and Rheumatism*, an article entitled, "Diet Therapy for Rheumatoid Arthritis," by Richard S. Panush et al., addresses this situation. The article states, " . . . little if any objective information about diet therapy for arthritis is available." As a result, a study was undertaken involving twenty-six patients. Eleven of the patients were placed on an experimental diet assumed to be beneficial for arthritis, and fifteen others were placed on a placebo diet. Although the results were not overwhelmingly conclusive, the article nevertheless states, "Five patients on the experimental diet improved an average of 32 percent."

The report went onto say that "Two patients on the experimental diet improved notably, elected to remain on the experimental diet following the study period and have continued to improve and note exacerbations of disease upon consuming non-experimental foods." Based on the results of the experiment, the article concludes, " . . . it seems reasonable to regard the notion that environmental or nutritional modifications might ameliorate arthritis as a provocative hypothesis requiring further experimentation."

In another article in the same issue, Dr. Morris Ziff commented on the dietary experiment concerning arthritis: "All things considered, there appears to be a case for the investigation of diet in the treatment of rheumatoid arthritis."

This initial dietary experiment represents an interesting and exciting first step in trying to discover whether diet and arthritis are linked. From this beginning it is apparent that further research needs to be conducted.

Another school of thought already strongly links arthritis to diet. This belief is occurring primarily among allergists. *Allergies* are a bodily reaction to food and other substances in the environment. A common allergic reaction occurs when we eat something and suddenly break out in a rash or experience itching or sneezing. These are short-term, or immediate reactions. However, many allergists believe that there are long-term reactions to the foods we eat. This fact is reflected in the following quote by James Breneman, M.D., who chaired a committee formed by the American College of Allergists.

"I do not think there is any doubt in many cases arthritis symptoms are linked to these delayed food allergies. A number of studies have shown that, and while we do not have precise figures on how common the problem is, I think it is reasonable to estimate in the neighborhood of 60 to 70 percent of arthritis suffers would benefit from dietary manipulation."

These allergists cite pork, wheat products, nightshades, milk, eggs, and alcohol as the most common offenders in delayed food reactions. As a result of their experiences, many allergists are recommending that arthritis patients restrict the intake of these foods.

In addition to the above findings, a growing number of individual practitioners are uncovering a link between diet and arthritis. A Chinese physician, Collin Dong, M.D., has discovered that avoiding the intake of red meat, dairy foods, and nightshades can be effective in helping many arthritis suffers. In his book, *New Hope for the Arthritic*, he cites allergic reaction along with chemical pollution of food as causes of arthritis. He proposes dietary change as a primary component in recovery from arthritis. And he recommends that dietary changes be long term for continuing recovery effects, otherwise arthritis may return if the causative foods are again included.

Dr. Norman Childers, Blake Professor of Horticulture at Rutgers University, has published a study about the connection between arthritis and the *nightshade* family. The nightshade vegetables include potato, tomato, pepper, and eggplant. Dr. Childers feels that these foods contain toxins that can cause arthritis, most notably in potato and tomato an alkaloid poison called *solanine* He has found that eliminating them helps diminish the symptoms of arthritis. He believes his own recovery from arthritis is the result of these dietary changes.

Other studies have linked overconsumption of dairy products with arthritis. In his book, *Don't Drink Your Milk*, Dr. Frank Oski documents some of the effects of excessive milk consumption. He cites a number of health problems that result from this practice, including rheumatoid arthritis.

## Conclusion

What can we conclude from the literature concerning arthritis and its causes?

- First, there is a host of biological phenomena in the body that are related to arthritis. These have generated a variety of theories concerning the cause of the disease. However, they have yet to provide a substantive answer that would result in an effective method for prevention or recovery.
- Second, there is a surprising lack of authoritative research on the relationship between diet and arthritis. On account of this we cannot dismiss the possibility of a link between diet and arthritis.
- Third, a growing body of literature suggests a connection between specific foods and arthritis.
- Fourth, in some individual cases it appears that dietary changes may help in recovering from arthritis.

As time goes by we are finding that food is much more a part of arthritis than was previously believed, and as this evidence continues to mount, the possibility of establishing a clear, comprehensive understanding of the role of diet in the development of arthritis is growing.

The macrobiotic point of view already recognizes that the fundamental aspect of a healthy lifestyle is diet, and the most important point in understanding arthritis is to realize how food affects us. In order to see why this is, we can begin by examining the principle behind the macrobiotic view of life and how to apply this principle to understand comprehensively our human body and why the macrobiotic approach to diet is basic common sense.

# 3. Arthritis and Diet

If we look carefully at the symptoms of arthritis, an overall pattern begins to emerge. Although varied and complex, these symptoms are manifestations of two basic tendencies.

In one, the joints become hard and stiff, and may become fused. In the other, they become swollen, enlarged, or inflammed. The first category is often accompanied by the following characteristics:

1.  Less general body involvement with fewer accompanying symptoms.
2.  Less inflammation.
3.  Less swelling.
4.  Slower, deeper pain.
5.  More involvement of the central and lower parts of the body.

In the second category, the following characteristics emerge:

1.  More general body involvement with more accompanying symptoms.
2.  More inflammation.
3.  A greater degree of swelling.
4.  More intense, cyclic pain.
5.  A greater involvement of more peripheral or upper areas of the body.

Understanding the overall pattern of arthritis is the first step toward understanding the cause of the disease. Our next question must be, "What creates these differences in the way arthritis develops?"

In macrobiotic thinking, our physical condition is recreated every day by what we take in from the environment. Of these, daily food and drink play a vital role. Every day, we internalize the environment in the form of food. We use the energy and nutrients in food to renew our bodies and provide energy for our life activities. Therefore, the quality of food and drink is primary in determining the  quality of our life, including the condition of our blood and body fluids, tissues and cells, and bones and joints.

Like the symptoms of arthritis, daily food can be understood in terms of two complementary tendencies. Certain foods produce expanding effects in the body, while others create contracting effects. These tendencies—which are found throughout nature—are referred to in macrobiotics as yin and yang.

For the most part, animal foods—including eggs, meat, hard cheese, poultry, and seafood—are more yang or contracting. When eaten excessively, they can produce an overly contracted state in the body. This condition can result in twisting and distortion of the joints. How these foods affect the body—which joints are affected, for instance, and to what degree, and whether other symptoms appear —depends on the individual's particular food choices. For example, someone may eat beef every day, while someone else may enjoy chicken and eggs. The amount of the food eaten and the proportion of other foods that are also included determines the particular set of symptoms that an individual experiences.

Dairy foods also affect the bones and joints. Certain dairy foods, including milk, butter, cream, ice cream, whipped cream, and yogurt produce more extreme expansive effects in the body. The fats they contain often accumulate in the upper part of the body, and con- tribute to symptoms such as swelling and inflammation. Other types of dairy food, including hard, salty cheeses, produce more contracting effects. The fats and minerals they contain tend to accumulate in the lower body, and contribute to tightening or hardening in the joints.

Overconsumption of foods such as these, which are high in satu- rated fat and cholesterol, affects other parts of the body as well. In the circulatory system, for example, the arteries and blood vessels —which are normally open and flexible—can easily become clogged with deposits of saturated fat and cholesterol. As the blood vessels become narrow and constricted, blood no longer flows smoothly through them. In some cases, the flow of blood to an organ or other part of the body can be cut off. When this happens in the blood vessels that supply the heart, the result is a heart attack. When it occurs in the vessels that supply the brain, the result is a stroke. Both conditions are common today because people eat a large volume of animal food. As we can see, overintake of these extremes creates imbalance in the body and leads to sickness.

Avoiding the extreme foods that lead to the development of atherosclerosis—and substituting low-fat foods such as whole grains, beans, and fresh vegetables—is a constructive and natural way to prevent heart disease. However, rather than making dietary changes, many people have turned to a more extreme, artificial method—daily doses of aspirin—in hopes of preventing these conditions. Aspirin is an extremely yin or expansive product that produces a wide range of side effects. Aspirin interferes with the capacity of the blood to clot, and therefore makes it harder for wounds to heal. It can also cause the blood vessels to expand and erupt, resulting in bleeding. Aspirin induced bleeding occurs often in the stomach, intestines, and other digestive organs.

As we have seen, many cardiovascular diseases result from over-consumption of animal foods that are high in saturated fat and cholesterol. Aspirin, a more extreme, expanding substance, can some-times slow the rate at which these deposits accumulate. However, it does not change the cause, and carries the risk of side effects. More-over, many cardiovascular conditions have an opposite dietary cause. They arise from overintake of sugar, coffee, soft drinks, milk, ice cream, tropical fruits, and other foods with more extreme yin, or expansive effects. A stroke caused by the eruption of blood vessels in the brain is an example of this type of disorder. As researchers have discovered, aspirin—an extremely expansive product—does not help these conditions, and in fact could make them worse.

In general, plant foods are more yin, or expanded than animal foods. However, there is a wide range of variation in their degree of expansiveness. Some vegetable foods, especially those grown in the tropics, are far more expansive than those grown in more temperate regions. Vegetables such as tomatoes, potatoes, sweet potatoes, yams, eggplant, peppers, and others that come from tropical or semi-tropical areas have more extreme yin effects, Tropical or semi-tropical fruits, including banana, pineapple, and citrus, are even more ex-pansive, as are products like coffee, sugar, chocolate, and spices. Among edible plants, those such as whole grains, beans, fresh locally grown vegetables, sea vegetables, and others that originate in a tem-perate zone have a more even balance of expanding and contracting, or yin and yang energies. A chart classifying major categories of food into yin and yang is presented below.

More extreme yin foods are also associated with the development of arthritis. For example, the role that vegetables such as potato, tomato, eggplant, and peppers play in arthritis is becoming increasing-ly recognized. In the book, *Arthritis and the Nightshades*, Dr. Norman Childers reports that once he removed these vegatables from his diet, he noticed an immediate improvement in his arthritis.

Potatoes and tomatoes originated in Central and South America. They were discovered by the Spanish during the 1600s and brought back to Europe. At first, they were regarded with suspicion by the general population. However, after a period of time, they were slowly accepted throughout Europe.

When potatoes were first cultivated in Europe, they produced an abundant crop. As a result, they were widely regarded throughout

**Fig. 7  Examples of Foods as Generally Classified by Yin and Yang**

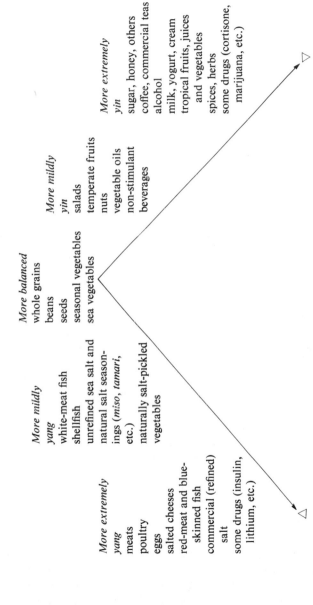

*More extremely yang*
meats
poultry
eggs
salted cheeses
red-meat and blue-skinned fish
commercial (refined) salt
some drugs (insulin, lithium, etc.)

*More mildly yang*
white-meat fish
shellfish
unrefined sea salt and natural salt seasonings (*miso, tamari,* etc.)
naturally salt-pickled vegetables

*More balanced*
whole grains
beans
seeds
seasonal vegetables
sea vegetables

*More mildly yin*
salads
temperate fruits
nuts
vegetable oils
non-stimulant beverages

*More extremely yin*
sugar, honey, others
coffee, commercial teas
alcohol
milk, yogurt, cream
tropical fruits, juices and vegetables
spices, herbs
some drugs (cortisone, marijuana, etc.)

the continent as a readily available source of nourishment. But because they were being grown in a very different environment from the one in which they originated, they were vulnerable to various blights and insects. As potatoes replaced the more hardy species of grains that had been cultivated on European soil for millennia, people grew increasingly dependent on them as a primary food. As a result, when blight struck the potato crop in Ireland in the 1840s, millions of people starved.

Potatoes and tomatoes contain a toxic molecule called *solanine*. This alkaloid poison is related to nicotine and caffeine, and is concentrated under the skin of the potato, in green spots, and in sprouts. Solanine adversely effects the digestive and nervous systems, and is increasingly suspected as playing an role in the development of arthritis.

Evidence is accumulating that these vegetables, which are members of the nightshade family, may deplete calcium from the bones and cause it to be deposited in the joints, blood vessels, and other parts of the body. Overintake of these foods may contribute to a weakening of the intestines, so that elimination of waste becomes less efficient. This accelerates the build up of toxins in and around the joints, as well as in other parts of the body. Excessive consumption of these foods can contribute to calcification, swelling, and inflammation in the joints.

Once, a woman came for macrobiotic advice. She was originally from Peru, which is where the potato originated. During her early life, she ate potatoes that were prepared according to traditional methods—including sun drying them, pounding them into a paste, and using them more as a condiment than as a main vegetable. However, once she moved north to the United States, she started eating potatoes every day as a main food. Her intake was much larger than it had been in Peru. Moreover, she began to eat them American-style, including baked and as French fries. This continued for many years, during which time her health began to deteriorate. By the time she came to one of our educational programs, most of the joints in her body were intensely painful and she was unable to have a bowel movement more than once a week, and then only with the help of enemas.

Refined sugar, another extreme product, also affects the bones and joints. Simple sugars, such as those found in honey, refined sugar, and maple syrup are quickly absorbed into the bloodstream, causing the blood to become overacidic. To compensate, the body's internal reserve of minerals is mobilized to create buffer reactions that neutralize and discharge these acids. If the intake of simple sugar is chronic, the supply of minerals in the bloodstream can become exhausted, at which time calcium in the bones and teeth may be utilized to balance the excessive intake of candy, soft drinks, and sugary desserts. In severe cases, bones can become brittle and start to erode as the person's stock of minerals continues to be depleted.

## Categories of Arthrits

In general, the symptoms of arthritis can be classified into two distinct categories, according to their underlying cause.

- *More Yin (Expansive) Arthritis:* Produced by excessive intake of more extreme yin foods and beverages, such as fruits, fruit juice—especially tropical and semi-tropical varieties—spices, stimulant and aromatic herbs and beverages, soft drinks, sugar, artificial sweeteners, honey, chocolate, and vinegars, as well as excessive intake of tomato, potato, eggplant, and other vegetables of tropical origin.

- *More Yang (Contractive) Arthritis:* Caused by an excessive intake of more extreme yang food categories, including meat, eggs, shellfish, and other animal foods. Large amounts of salt and other minerals, including the excessive intake of calcium associated with the regular consumption of dairy foods, also creates a more contractive condition in the joints.

Despite these differences, however, the types of arthritis in either category are aggravated to varying degrees by the consumption of excessive oil and fat from either animal or vegetable sources. In addition, both types are accelerated by excessive intake of liquid in general, and of icy cold drinks such as soda, beer, and alcoholic drinks, and other cold beverages. Ice cream is of course one of the major contributing factors.

More than one-hundred varieties of arthritis have been identified so far. However, they can all be classified into either more yin or more yang categories (some represent combinations of both extremes) according to their cause and the nature of the symptoms they create. Further, we can divide these two major categories into subcategories according to the degree of more yin (expansive) or more yang (contractive) symptoms displayed. This classification corresponds to the understanding of energy trasnformation that underlies the traditional practice of acupuncture and other forms of Oriental medicine, as well as the modern practice of the macrobiotic way of eating.

In the traditional macrobiotic view, yin and yang appear in the continual movement or cycling of energy that occurs throughout nature. (The term "energy" is used in this context to describe all phenomena, and not just invisible radiation or waves.) Everything, even the most dense metal or the hardest gemstone, the diamond, is vibrating at the atomic level. Moreover, all things eventually change their state or form; nothing in this universe is static or unchanging.

On the earth, the cycling of yin and yang is revealed in night and day, and in the changing of the seasons. During cold winter months, for example, energy in the atmosphere becomes more condensed. Plants and animals are dormant and inactive, while human activity becomes more inwardly focused. During the warm summer months, more expansive energy prevails in nature. Plants become more lush and abundant, and people become more active and outgoing.

Similarly, at night, the energy in the atmosphere becomes more still, quiet, and downward moving; while in the morning and during the day, it becomes brighter, more active, and upward moving.

In this cycle, energy moves back and forth between expansion and contraction, warm and cold temperatures, and brightness and darkness with varying stages of both tendencies in between. Spring, for example, represents the beginning of expansion. New vegetation appears in the spring and green (a more yin color) begins to predominate. Summer is the period of peak expansion, as higher temperatures stimulate abundant growth in the vegetable world. Then, energy begins to change around the time of the autumnal equinox. During this period, known in the Orient as late summer (or in America as Indian summer), we begin moving toward a period of greater downward, or contracting energy.

Contracting energy reaches a peak during the autumn, as trees and other forms of vegetation shed their leaves and return to a dormant state. After the winter solstice, the sun's energy slowly reactivates energy in the atmosphere and in the vegetable kingdom. This gradual process is somewhat offset by the continuing cold temperatures of winter, so that energy in the atmosphere tends to float between expansion and contraction, or upward and downward movement.

Similar patterns occur in the cycle of day and night, and throughout nature. Throughout history, a variety fo names were used to describe the stages in this cycle. The names used in macrobiotic thinking describe the predominant direction in which energy is moving at each stage in the cycle. In macrobiotics, the stages of energy transformation are referred to as: (1) "upward" energy (spring); (2) "active" or "expansive" energy (summer); (3) "downward" energy (late summer); (4) "condensed" energy (autumn); and (5) "floating" energy (winter). Traditional Oriental doctors associated these stages with natural phenomena, and named them: (1) "tree" nature; (2) "fire" nature; (3) "soil" nature; (4) "metal" nature; and (5) "water" nature.

Table 2    The Five Transformations of Energy

|  | A | B | C | D | E |
|---|---|---|---|---|---|
| Energy: | Upward | Very active | Downward | Solidified | Floating |
| Examples: | Gas | Plasma | Condensation | Solid | Liquid |
|  | Tree | Fire | Soil | Metal | Water |
| Organ Energy: | Liver, gall bladder | Heart, small intestine | Spleen-pancreas, stomach | Lungs, large intestine | kidneys, bladder |
| Direction: | East | South | Center | West | North |
| Season: | Spring | Summer | Late summer | Autumn | Winter |
| Time of month: | Increasing half-moon | Full moon | Obscured moon | Decreasing half-moon | New moon |
| Time of day: | Morning | Noon | Afternoon | Evening | Night |
| Environment: | Windy | Hot | Humid | Dry | Cold |
| Grain: | Wheat, barley | Corn | Millet | Rice | Beans |
| Vegetables: | Sprouts and upward-growing plants | Enlarged leafy plants | Round plants | Contracted, small plants | Root plants |
| Fruits: | Spring fruits | Summer fruits | Late summer fruits | Autumn fruits | Winter and dried fruits |
| Odor: | Oily, greasy | Burning | Fragrant | Fishy | Putrefying |
| Tastes: | Sour | Bitter | Sweet | Pungent | Salty |
| Physical parts: | Tissues | Blood vessels | Muscles | Skin | Bones |
| Physical branches: | Nails | Body hair and facial color | Breast, lips | Breath | Head hair |
| Skin color: | Blue, gray | Red | Yellow, milky | Pale | Black, dark |
| Physical liquids: | Tears | Sweat | Slaver | Snivel | Saliva |
| Physical changes: | Gripping | Anxious | Sobbing | Coughing | Shivering |
| 5 Voices: | Shouting | Talking | Singing | Crying | Groaning |
| 5 Functions: | Color | Odor | Taste | Voice | Fluid |
| Psychological reaction: | Anger, excitement | Laughing, talkative | Indecisive, suspicious | Sadness, depression | Fear, insecurity |

This classification can be extended to all things in the natural world. As we can see in the Table 2, among vegetables, certain varieties, such as root vegetables, have more downward or condensed energy. Others, such as sprouts and large leafy greens, grow in an upward direction and are more expanded. Still others, especially round vegetables like cabbage and onions, are somewhat in between. Similar distinctions can be found among cereal grains, fruits, and other categories of food.

Different parts of the body, such as the internal organs, can also be classified according to their energy quality. This view, in which everything is seen as a manifestation of energy, is not new. It was recorded in the *Nei-Ching*, or *Yellow Emperor's Classic of Internal Medicine*, the book that first described the theoretical foundations of Oriental medicine thousands of years ago. (For additional details concerning the stages of energy transformation and other cycles of energy, readers are referred to *Macrobiotics and Oriental Medicine*, by Michio Kushi, with Phillip Jannetta, Japan Publications, 198.)

Arthritis represents an imbalance in the flow of nutrients and energy in the body. Thus, an understanding of yin and yang and the stages of energy transformation can help solve the mystery of arthritis. For example, joints that become hard, stiff, or fused are examples of an excess of contracting, or downward energy. The greater the extent to which these symptoms appear, the greater the degree of contracting energy the condition represents. On the other hand, joints that become swollen, enlarged, or inflamed are examples of an excess of upward, or expanding energy. The greater the extent to which these symptoms appear, or the more of them there are, the greater the degree of expanding energy the arthritis represents.

### Fig. 8 Symptoms of Arthritis and the Stages of Energy

| *More Yin* | *More Yang* |
| --- | --- |
| More general body involvement | Less general body involvement |
| More accompanying symptoms | Fewer accompanying symptoms |
| More inflammation | Less inflammation |
| More swelling | Less swelling |
| More intense, cyclic pain | Slower, deeper pain |
| Peripheral joints affected more | Central joints affected more |

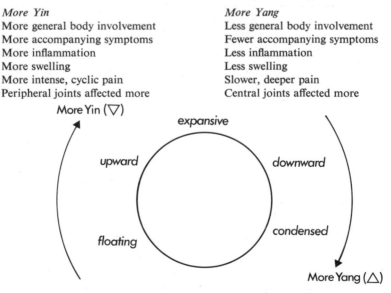

In Figure 8, the primary symptoms mentioned at the beginning of the chapter are correlated with the expanding and contracting movement of energy. Let us now see how the major types of arthritis correlate with these stages of energy transformation.

*Rheumatoid Arthritis.*   The primary symptoms of rheumatoid arthritis are swelling and inflammation in the joints and intense cyclic pain that can become chronic. The most commonly affected joints are the knuckles, wrists, knees, and balls of the feet.

This type of arthritis is often accompanied by a variety of symptoms such as low fever, fatigue, loss of appetite and weight, and anemia, as well as by possible pleurisy, enlargement of the spleen, tachycardia, and the development of rheumatoid nodules (lumps that form under the skin), especially near the elbow.

The involvement of more peripherally located joints in the hands, legs, and feet, combined with inflammation and a large number of accompanying symptoms, indicates that rheumatoid arthritis arises from an excess of upward energy in the body. The overintake of foods with strong expanding energy, such as fruit and fruit juices (especially tropical or semi-tropical varieties), spices, concentrated sweeteners, alcohol, and vegetables such as tomato, potato, and eggplant, is a primary cause of this condition. The overconsumption of fats, including those in milk, ice cream, butter, cheese, chicken, and eggs, can also contribute to the accumulation of upward energy that leads to rheumatoid arthritis.

*Lupus and Arthritis.*   The primary symptoms of the arthritis that occurs in lupus include joint pain and tenderness on motion, but without swelling or inflammation. Joints that are most often affected are the wrists, knuckles (especially of the middle fingers), and the knees.

This condition is part of a wide range of symptoms that involve the body. Skin rashes, especially over the cheeks and bridge of the nose, hair loss, *photosensitivity* (adverse skin reactions to sunlight), mouth ulcers, excessive loss of protein in the urine, inflammation around the heart, of the pleural lining, and of the membrane surrounding the abdominal cavity, depressed blood counts, and psychosis or convulsions can occur in lupus.

The pattern of joint involvement is generally the same as in rheumatoid arthritis. Even though the joints do not swell, the large number of accompanying symptoms—much greater in lupus than in rheumatoid arthritis—indicate that lupus is a more extremely expansive condition.

Lupus is caused primarily by the overintake of powerfully yin foods such as sugar, artificial sweeteners, tropical fruits, ice cream, chocolate, soft drinks, chemicals, drugs, medications, and vegetables with a tropical origin. Animal fats and proteins, including those in milk and other dairy products, also contribute by causing mucus and fat to accumulate in the lungs, kidneys, and intestines, thereby diminishing the body's ability to discharge toxins.

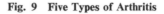

**Fig. 9    Five Types of Arthritis**

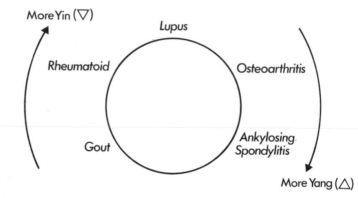

*Osteoarthritis.*   The major symptoms of osteoarthritis include erosion of the cartilage in the joints, so that the joint space narrows, and development of bony growths that cause the bones to fuse. The hip, spine, knee, and foot joints are commonly affected, while hard nodes often form in the last joints of the fingers. Generally, there are no accompanying symptoms.

As we can see, the joints in the central or lower body—especially the hips and spine—are often affected, with some involvement of the more peripherally located joints in the knees, feet, and fingers. The location of these joints, plus the contracting nature of the symptoms, indicate that this is primarily a condition in which downward, or contracting energy becomes excessive.

Foods that accelerate contracting energy include animal fats, such as those in meat, eggs, poultry, and cheese, as well as excessive amounts of salt and other minerals. The hard, saturated fats in animal foods tend to gather in the joints located deeper or further down in the body. The development of nodes on the end joints of the fingers is also a sign of overconsumption of fats, especially those in chicken, eggs, and poultry. Fruits, sugar, concentrated sweeteners, tropical fruits and vegetables, and more extreme yin foods also contribute to the gradual erosion of the joints seen in osteoarthrits.

*Ankylosing Spondylitis.* This disease produces inflammation where a tendon or ligament attaches to the bone, resulting in fusion of the joint. It begins in the lower spine and moves upward, and can be accompanied by minor fatigue, weight loss, and inflammation of the aortic valve of the heart.

The pattern of ankylosing spondylitis shows that the joints of the lower spine are affected first. In other words, it begins in the lower, central part of the body. There is no peripheral joint involvement. Ankylosing spondylitis is caused primarily by excessive condensed energy, resulting from overconsumtion of meat, eggs, chicken, hard cheese and other dairy fats, salt and other minerals, and baked flour products.

Overconsumption of strong contracting foods can cause twisting and distortion of the human structure and eventual fusion of the spinal joints. Moreover, a diet high in animal fats adversely affects the heart, as it does in ankylosing spondylitis. In extreme cases, the person's spine is stiffly bent forward with the head tilted at an angle to the body, a condition that can result from the overintake of chicken and eggs. The rigidity of the lower part of the spine is related to problems in the opposite, frontal areas of the body, including the bladder, sexual organs, and intestines.

Excessive intake of sugar, soft drinks, tropical fruits and vegetables, spices, and other foods with more extreme expanding energy contributes to swelling and inflammation in the regions where tendons and ligaments attach to the bones, as well as in the aortic valve.

*Gout.* Gout produces painful swelling and inflammation in the base of the large toe, as well as in the instep, ankles, knees, wrists, and fingers. It is often accompanied by kidney stones.

The pattern of gout shows that the peripheral joints of the lower region of the body are most affected, predominately the base of the large toe. Painful attacks, accompanied by swelling and inflammation, occur mostly at night and are cyclic in nature. Gout is an example of an excess of both expanding and contracting extremes, and is classified in the category that corresponds to "floating" energy. Gout results from excessive consumption of extreme combinations such as meat and alcohol, cheese and wine, meat with heavy sauces and gravies followed by rich sugary desserts, and barbecued meats followed by iced drinks.

## The Progressive Development of Arthritis ——————

Arthritis is part of a degenerative process that normally develops over time. As we can see, it is rooted in our daily diet and way of life. The risk of developing it increases as we get older.

Healthy children have a condition that is the opposite of arthirtis. Their bodies are flexible, and they are active and energetic. Arthritis represents an unnatural form of aging, with the body becoming stiff and rigid. However, if our diet and way of life are balanced throughout life, arthritis need not occur, even in old age.

When our diet is based around more centrally balanced foods, such as whole cereal grains, beans, fresh local vegetables, low-fat seafood, local fruits, and others, the body is able to discharge the waste products of digestion and metabolism through normal processes such as daily bowel movement and urination, perspiration, breathing, daily activity, and, in women, through menstruation. However, if our diet is more extreme, including frequent consumption of foods from either category, normal channels of elimination are not able to discharge the excessive factors they contain. When this happens, abnormal discharge mechanisms are called into play, including symptoms such as coughing, diarrhea, sneezing, and allergic reactions. Periodic colds and flu are also the body's attempt to discharge the toxins that build up after a certain period of unbalanced eating.

If our diet continues on a more extreme course, however, even periodic discharges are not enough to rid the body of toxic overload. At this point, excess begins to accumulate—usually in the form of fat and mucus—in parts of the body that have a direct channel to the outside, such as the sinuses, lungs, breasts, kidneys, intestines, and the reproductive organs, including the uterus, ovaries, and prostate gland. A hard layer of fat may also accumulate just below the skin. If the diet remains extreme, conditions such as severe sinus blockage, breast cysts, chronic coughing and chest congestion, kidney stones, intestinal polyps, ovarian cysts, fibroid tumors, and enlargement of the prostate may develop. Hard, dry skin is a sign that fat has also built up below the surface of the body.

When the intake of extremes continues beyond this stage, excess begins to accumulate deeper in the body, including the arteries and blood vessels, and in organs such as the heart, liver, spleen, and pancreas. At this stage, excess is often deposited in and around the joints, causing the degenerative changes that result in arthritis.

The volume and quality of excess determines when, where, and how the joints are affected. Arthritis is not an isolated condition, but part of a process that involves the entire body. By the time degenerative changes appear in the joints, parallel accumulations have also developed in the internal organs, causing their functions to diminish. For example, many people with arthritis suffer from a wide range of degenerative conditions such as high blood pressure, obesity, hardening of the arteries, diabetes, various types of heart disease, and cancer. Arthritis is just one among many symptoms of body-wide deterioration resulting from an unbalanced diet and way of life.

Today, this process begins at an early age. Researchers have already discovered fatty streaks in the arteries of kindergarten children. Moreover, a shockingly high percentage of American children are overweight, an indication that the buildup of fats and other excessive factors is already underway. At the same time, many children and young people experience stiffness in the joints. Young people in modern nations are often less flexible than adults in cultures where the modern diet has not penetrated. In this sense, many people in the modern world have become unnaturally old before their time.

# 4. The Macrobiotic Approach ▬▬▬

As we have seen, a properly balanced diet can play a primary role in lowering the risk of arthritis. Let us now review the outlines of the Standard Macrobiotic Diet. This way of eating, with appropriate modifications for each individual, can serve as the basis for a more healthful and preventive lifestyle. By basing daily diet around more centrally balanced foods, such as whole cereal grains, beans, fresh local vegetables, sea vegetables, and others, the extremes that lead to accumulation of excess throughout the body—including the joints—can be minimized or avoided.

Macrobiotics offers more than just an orderly way of eating. It encompasses a whole lifestyle that respects human tradition and the order of nature, with the spirit of fostering personal and social well-being and creating a healthy and peaceful world.

In contrast to modern dietary habits, macrobiotic eating is based on the following nutritional considerations:

1. More centrally balanced complex carbohydrates and fewer simple sugars;
2. More vegetable-quality protein and less protein from animal sources;
3. Less overall consumption of fat—more unsaturated fat and less saturated fat;
4. Adequate consideration of the ideal balance between vitamins, minerals, and other nutritional factors;
5. Use of more organically grown, natural-quality food, and fewer chemically sprayed or fertilized items;
6. Use of more traditionally processed foods and fewer artifically and chemically processed foods;
7. A larger intake of foods in their whole form and less intake of refined and partial foods;
8. More consumption of foods rich in natural fiber rather than foods that have been devitalized.

These basic guidelines have been practiced daily for more than twenty years by hundreds of thousands of people throughout the world, including many families. Moreover, similar dietary practices have been observed traditionally by many cultures for thousands of years.

The guidelines in this chapter are designed for people living in temperate climates. Modifications are required if one lives in a tropical or subtropical climate, or a polar or semi-polar region. We also need to adjust our diet when we travel or move to one of these regions. It is also important to flexibly adapt these guidelines to suit everyone's individual needs and condition. For this reason, it is a good idea to meet with a qualified macrobiotic teacher or to participate in programs such as the *Macrobiotic Way of Life Seminar* presented by the Kushi Foundation in Boston, in order to receive individual guidance. (A schedule of these ongoing programs is available from the Kushi Foundation.)

## Standard Macrobiotic Way of Eating ━━━━━━━━

The guidelines that follow are broad and flexible. The standard macrobiotic way of eating offers an incredible variety of foods and cooking methods to choose from. You can apply them when selecting the highest quality natural foods for yourself and your family.

### Whole Grains

Within the standard macrobiotic way of eating and especially in a temperate climate, whole grains are an essential part of the daily diet. They comprise 40 to 60 percent (average 50 percent) of daily food intake.

*Kinds of Whole Grains and Grain Products*
*Brown Rice*
    Brown rice—short, medium, and long grain
    Genuine brown rice cream
    Puffed brown rice
    Brown rice flour products
    Brown rice flakes
*Sweet Brown Rice*
    Sweet brown rice grain
    *Mochi* (pounded sweet brown rice)
    Sweet brown rice flour products
*Wild Rice*
    Wild rice grain
*Whole Wheat*
    Whole wheat berries
    Whole wheat bread
    Whole wheat chapatis

50

## Fig. 10 Standard Macrobiotic Diet

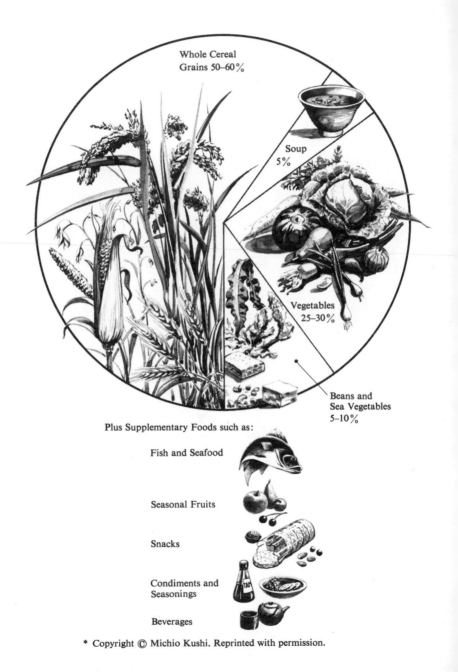

Whole Cereal
Grains 50–60%

Soup
5%

Vegetables
25–30%

Beans and
Sea Vegetables
5–10%

Plus Supplementary Foods such as:

Fish and Seafood

Seasonal Fruits

Snacks

Condiments and
Seasonings

Beverages

Whole wheat noodles and pasta
Whole wheat flakes
Whole wheat flour products, such as crackers, matzos, muffins, and others
Couscous
Bulgur
*Fu* (baked puffed wheat gluten)
*Seitan* (wheat gluten)
*Barley*
Barley grain
Pearl barley
Pearled barley
Puffed barley
Barley flour products
*Rye*
Rye grain
Rye bread
Rye flakes
Rye flour products
*Millet*
Millet grain
Millet flour products
Puffed millet
*Oats*
Whole oats
Steel-cut oats
Rolled oats
Oatmeal
Oat flakes
Oat flour products and puffed oats
*Corn*
Corn on the cob
Corn grits
Corn meal
*Arepas*
Corn flour products such as corn bread, muffins, etc.
Puffed corn
Popped corn
*Buckwheat*
Buckwheat groats
Buckwheat noodles and pasta
Buckwheat flour products such as pancakes, etc.

Cooked whole grains are preferable to flour products or to cracked or rolled grains because of easier digestibility. In general, it is better to keep intake of flour products—or cracked or rolled grains—to less than 15 to 20 percent of your daily whole grain intake.

## Soups

Soups may comprise about 5 percent of each person's daily intake. For most people, that averages out to about one or two cups or small bowls of soup per day, depending on individual desire and preference. Soups can include vegetables, grains, beans, sea vegetables, noodles or other grain products, bean products like tofu, tempeh, and others, or, occasionally, fish or seafood. Soups can be moderately seasoned with either miso, tamari soy sauce, sea salt, umeboshi plum or paste, or occasional ginger.

Soups can be made thick and rich, or as simple clear broths. Vegetable, grain, or bean stews can also be enjoyed, while a variety of garnishes, such as scallions, parsley, *nori* sea vegetable, and croutons may be used to enhance the appearance and flavor of soups.

## Vegetables

A wide selection of vegetable dishes prepared in a variety of cooking styles may comprise approximately 30 percent of daily food intake.

| *Kinds of Vegetables* | *Daikon* | Mushrooms |
|---|---|---|
| Acorn squash | Daikon greens | Mustard greens |
| Bok choy | Dandelion leaves | Onion |
| Broccoli | Dandelion roots | Parsley |
| Burdock root | Endive | Parsnip |
| Buttercup squash | Escarole | Pumpkin |
| Butternut squash | Green beans | Patty pan squash |
| Cabbage | Green peas | Radish |
| Celery | Hokkaido pumpkin | Red cabbage |
| Celery root | Hubbard squash | Romaine lettuce |
| Carrots | Iceberg lettuce | Scallions |
| Carrot tops | *Jinenjo* | *Shiitake* mushrooms |
| Cauliflower | Jerusalem artichoke | Snap beans |
| Chinese cabbage | Kale | Summer squash |
| Chives | Kohlrabi | Turnip greens |
| Collard greens | Leeks | Watercress |
| Coltsfoot | Lotus root | Wax beans |
| Cucumber | Lamb's-quarters | |

Vegetables can be served in soups, or with grains, beans, or sea vegetables. They can also be used in making rice rolls (macrobiotic *sushi*), served with noodles or pasta, cooked with fish, or served alone. The methods for cooking vegetables that are introduced in this book include boiling, steaming, pressing, sautéing (both waterless and with oil), and pickling. A variety of natural seasonings, including miso, tamari soy sauce, sea salt, and brown rice or umeboshi vinegar are recommended in vegetable cookery.

**Beans**

The standard macrobiotic way of eating recommends regular consumption of beans and bean products. Beans may comprise 5 to 10 percent of daily food intake.

*Kinds of Beans*

| | |
|---|---|
| *Azuki* beans | Navy beans |
| Black-eyed peas | Pinto beans |
| Black turtle beans | Soybeans |
| Black soybeans | Split peas |
| Chick-peas (garbanzo beans) | Whole dried peas |
| Great northern beans | Bean sprouts |
| Kidney beans | Other beans which have |
| Lentils | been traditionally used |
| Lima beans | |
| Mung beans | |

*Kinds of Bean Products*
   Dried *tofu* (soybean curd that has been dried)
   Fresh tofu
   *Okara* (residue in making tofu)
   *Natto* (fermented soybeans)
   *Tempeh* (fermented soybeans)

Beans and bean products are more easily digested when cooked with a small volume of seasoning such as sea salt, miso, or kombu sea vegetable. They may also be prepared with vegetables, chestnuts, dried apples, or raisins, or occasionally sweetened with grain sweeteners like barley malt and rice honey. Beans and bean products may be served in soups and side dishes, or cooked with grains or sea vegetables.

## Sea Vegetables

Sea vegetables may be used daily in cooking. Side dishes can be made with *arame* or *hijiki* and included several times per week. Wakame and kombu can be used daily in miso and other soups, in vegetable and bean dishes, or as condiments. Toasted nori is also recommended for daily or regular use, while agar-agar can be used from time to time in making a natural jelled dessert known as *kanten* (agar-agar also has natural laxative properties). Below is a list of the sea vegetables for use in macrobiotic cooking:

*Kinds of Sea Vegetables*
  Arame
  Agar-agar
  Dulse
  *Hijiki*
  Irish moss (sea moss)

Kombu
*Mekabu*
*Nekabu*
*Nori*
Wakame

## Fish and Seafood

The standard macrobiotic way of eating recommends fish and seafood as an occasional supplement to the above categories of food—grains, soups, vegetables, beans, and beverages. The amount of fish or seafood can vary according to personal needs and can range from once in a while to several times a week. The average, however, is twice or three times a week—with the amount not exceeding 20 percent of the total volume of food consumed that day. The kinds of fish and seafood recommended are those with less saturated fat and those which are most easily digested.

*Kinds of Fish and Seafood*
  Carp
  Cod
  Dried fish
  Small dried fish (*iriko*)
  Flounder
  Haddock
  Halibut

Herring
Scrod
Smelt
Snapper
Sole
Trout
White-meat fish

*Seafood Used Occasionally*
  Cherrystone clams
  Littleneck clams
  Clams
  Crab

Octopus
Oysters
Lobster
Shrimp

*Infrequently Used Fish,* not preferred for regular use

| | |
|---|---|
| Bluefish | Tuna |
| Salmon | Other blue-skinned or red-meat |
| Sardines | fish |
| Swordfish | |

Garnishes are especially important in balancing fish and seafood. Recommended garnishes include: chopped scallions or parsley, grated raw daikon, ginger, radish or horseradish, green mustard paste (*wasabi*), raw salad, and shredded daikon.

## Fruit

The standard macrobiotic way of eating includes occasional consumption of fruit, depending upon climate, season, personal need, and circumstances. All traditionally used and commonly consumed fruits growing in a temperate climate are included. The regular use of tropical fruits in a temperate climate is not recommended.

*Kinds of Fruit*

| | |
|---|---|
| Apples | Persimmon |
| Apricots | Peaches |
| Blackberries | Plums |
| Cantaloupe | Raisins |
| Grapes | Raspberries |
| Grapefruit | Strawberries |
| Honeydew melon | Tangerines |
| Lemons | Watermelon |
| Mulberries | Wild berries |
| Oranges | |

## Pickles

Pickles can be eaten frequently as a supplement to main dishes. They stimulate appetite and help digestion. Some varieties—such as pickled daikon, or *takuan*—can be bought prepackaged in natural food stores. Other—such as quick pickles—can be prepared at home. Certain varieties take just a few hours to prepare, while others require more time.

A wide variety of pickles are fine for regular use, including salt, salt brine, bran, miso, tamari, umeboshi vinegar, and others. Sauerkraut may also be used in small volume on a regular basis.

**Seeds and Nuts**

Seeds and nuts can be eaten from time to time as snacks and garnishes. They can be roasted with or without sea salt, sweetened with barley or rice malt, or seasoned with tamari soy sauce. Seeds and nuts can be ground into butter, shaved and served as a topping, garnish, or ingredient in various dishes, including dessert. Below are varieties that can be used.

*Kinds of Nuts*
Almonds
Chestnuts
Filberts
Peanuts
*Less Frequently Used Nuts*
Brazil nuts
Cashews
Macadamia nuts

Pecans
Pinenuts
Small Spanish nuts
Walnuts

Other traditionally used nuts

*Kinds of Seeds*
Alfalfa seeds
Black sesame seeds
Poppy seeds
Pumpkin seeds
Squash seeds

Sunflower seeds
Umeboshi plum seeds
White sesame seeds
Others

**Snacks**

A variety of natural snacks may be enjoyed from time to time, including those made from whole grains, like cookies, bread, puffed cereals, mochi (pounded sweet brown rice), rice cakes, rice balls, and macrobiotic sushi. Nuts and seeds may also be used as snacks, for example by roasting them with sea salt, tamari soy sauce, or sweetening them with grain-based sweeteners.

**Condiments**

A variety of condiments may be used, some daily and others occasionally. Small amounts can be sprinkled on foods to adjust taste and nutritional value, and to stimulate appetite. They can be used on grains, soups, vegetables, beans, and sometimes desserts. The most frequently used varieties include:

*Gomashio* (roasted sesame seeds and sea salt)
Sea vegetable powders (with or without roasted sesame seeds)
*Tekka* (a special condiment made with soybean miso, sesame oil, burdock, lotus root, carrots, and ginger)
Umeboshi (pickled salt) plums
*Condiments that can be used occasionally:*
  Roasted sesame seeds
  Roasted and chopped *shiso* (pickled beefsteak plant) leaves
  *Shio kombu* (kombu cooked with tamari soy sauce and water)

Green nori flakes
Cooked nori condiment
Cooked miso with scallions or onions
Umeboshi or brown rice vinegar

**Seasonings**

A variety of seasonings can be used when cooking macrobiotically. It is better to avoid strong spicy seasonings such as curry, hot pepper, and others, and to use those which are naturally processed from vegetable products or natural sea salt, and which have been in use as a part of traditional diets. A list of seasonings is presented below:

*Kinds of Seasonings*

| | |
|---|---|
| Unrefined sea salt | Lemon juice |
| Soy sauce | Tangerine juice |
| Tamari soy sauce | Orange juice |
| Miso | Green mustard paste |
| Brown rice vinegar | Yellow mustard paste |
| Umeboshi vinegar | Sesame oil |
| Barley malt | Corn oil |
| Rice malt | Safflower oil |
| Grated ginger root | Mustard seed oil |
| Grated daikon | Olive oil |
| Grated radish | |
| Umeboshi paste | |
| Umeboshi plum | |

*Mirin* (sweet cooking wine)
*Amazaké* (fermented sweet brown rice beverage)
Other natural seasonings which have been traditionally used

## Garnishes

A variety of garnishes can be used to create balance among dishes and facilitate digestion. The use of garnishes depends upon the needs and desire of each person. The following garnishes can be used:

Grated daikon (for fish, mochi, noodles, and other dishes)
Grated radish (used like grated daikon)
Grated horseradish (used mostly for fish and seafood)
Chopped scallions (for noodles, fish and seafood, and so on)
Parsley
Lemon, tangerine, and orange slices (mainly for fish and seafood)
Others

## Desserts

A variety of natural desserts may be eaten from time to time, usually at the end of the main meal. Desserts can be made from azuki beans (sweetened with grain syrup, chestnuts, squash, or raisins); cooked or dried fruit; agar-agar (natural sea vegetable gelatin); grains (e.g., rice pudding, couscous cake, Indian pudding, etc.); and flour products (e.g., cookies, cakes, pies, muffins, etc., prepared with fruit or grain sweeteners).

## Beverages

A variety of beverages may be consumed daily or occasionally. Amounts can vary according to each person's needs and weather conditions. The beverages listed below can be used to comfortably satisfy the desire for liquid.

*Bancha* twig and stem tea
Roasted brown rice or barley tea
Cereal grain coffee
Spring or well water
Amazaké
Dandelion tea
Soybean milk (prepared with kombu)
Kombu tea
Lotus root tea
*Mu* tea
Other traditional non-stimulant and nonaromatic natural herbal beverages

*Saké* (fermented rice wine, without chemicals or sugar)
Beer (more natural quality)
Apple, grape, and apricot juice
Apple cider
Carrot, celery, and other vegetable juices

**Additional Foods**

In some cases, the standard macrobiotic diet can be temporarily
modified to include other foods. These modifications can be made
according to individual requirements and necessity; though within
usual practice, additional foods are usually not necessary for the
maintenance of health and well-being.

## Suggestions for Healthy Living ━━━━━━

Together with eating well, there are a number of practices that we
recommend for a healthier and more natural life. Practices such as
keeping physically active and using natural cooking utensils, fabrics,
and materials in the home are especially recommended. In the past,
people lived more closely with nature and ate a more balanced,
natural diet. With each generation, we have gotten further and further
from our roots in nature, and have experienced a corresponding
increase in cancer and other chronic illnesses.

The suggestions presented below complement a balanced natural
diet and can help everyone enjoy more satisfying and harmonious
living.

- Live each day happily without being preoccupied with your health,
  and try to keep mentally and physically active.
- View everything and everyone you meet with gratitude, particularly
  offering thanks before and after every meal.
- Please chew your food very well, at least 50 times per mouthful or
  until it becomes a liquid.
- It is best to retire before midnight and get up early every morning.
- It is best to avoid wearing synthetic or woolen clothing directly on
  the skin. As much as possible, wear cotton, especially for undergar-
  ments. Avoid excessive metallic accessories on the fingers, wrists,
  or neck. Keep such ornaments simple and graceful.
- If your strength permits, go outdoors in simple clothing. Walk on
  the grass, beach, or soil up to one-half hour every day. Keep your
  home in good order, from the kitchen, bathroom, bedroom, and
  living room, to every corner of the house.

- Initiate and maintain an active correspondence, extending your best wishes to parents, children, brothers and sisters, teachers and friends.
- Avoid taking long hot baths or showers unless you have been consuming too much salt or animal food.
- Scrub your entire body with a hot damp towel until the skin becomes red every morning or every night before retiring. If that is not possible, at least scrub your hands, feet, fingers, and toes.
- Avoid chemically perfumed cosmetics. For care of teeth, brush with natural preparations or sea salt.
- If your condition permits, exercise regularly as part of daily life, including activities like scrubbing floors, cleaning windows, and washing clothes. You may also participate in exercise programs such as yoga, martial arts, dance, or sports.
- Avoid using electric cooking devices (ovens and ranges) or microwave ovens. Convert to gas or wood-stove cooking at the earliest opportunity.
- It is best to minimize the use of color television and computer display units.
- Include some large green plants in your house to freshen and enrich the oxygen content of the air of your home.

The way in which we eat can be just as important as the choice of foods. Regular meals are better, and be sure to include a whole grain dish at each meal (the word "meal" actually means "crushed whole grain"). The amount of food eaten depends on each person's needs. Snacking is best kept moderate, so that it does not replace meals, while tea and other beverages can be enjoyed throughout the day as desired. Chewing is also important; try to chew each mouthful of food until it becomes liquid. You can eat whenever you feel hungry, but try to avoid eating before bedtime, preferably for three hours, except in unusual circumstances. Finally, learn to appreciate your foods and the health-giving properties they contain. Let your gratitude overflow to include nature, the universe, and all of the people with whom you share this wonderful life on earth.

# 5. Adjustments for Arthritis ━━━━━

In Chapter 4 we looked at the Standard Macrobiotic Diet in general: this is enough to prevent many cases of arthritis from developing, and can serve as the foundation for continuing health. However, in cases where arthritis already exists, it is necessary to make additional adjustments in this general dietary plan, to be followed for several months or until the condition improves, after which, the more general standard dietary approach may be adopted.

Both yin and yang varieties of arthritis reflect a basic extremism or imbalance in the body as a whole; so it is important in either case to avoid one-sided eating. Try to present a balanced mix of both energies at each meal, and try to cultivate a keen sense of balance in the aesthetic aspects of your cooking, such as complementing contrasting colors, textures, and tastes.

## General Recommendations for Arthritis ━━━━

1.   Extreme categories of both yin and yang foods are best avoided; in general, stay within the guidelines of the Standard Macrobiotic Diet. It is preferable to eat cooked foods only, although up to one-third of your vegetables may be lightly or quickly cooked. The consumption of both animal food and fruit is best kept to a minimum, and the use of salt, miso, tamari soy sauce, and other salty seasonings or condiments is best kept moderate.

2.   When selecting vegetables, it is advisable to avoid potatoes, tomatoes, eggplant, spinach, asparagus, avocados, beets, zucchini, and mushrooms (with the exception of shiitake). The main food in the daily diet can be whole grains, while supplemental foods may include cooked vegetables, beans, sea vegetables, and if desired, small portions of animal food such as fish and seafood, and an occasional small volume of cooked or dried fruit.

3.   As a special therapeutic dish, cook dried, shredded daikon with kombu and light tamari soy sauce to taste. Miso and scallions cooked together with several drops of seasme oil are also beneficial when used occasionally as a condiment.

4.   The use of wild vegetables such as fresh dandelion, watercress,

and others can also be helpful. Prepare them by first sautéing with a small amount of sesame oil, then adding a little water and simmering.

5.    Arthritis is commonly accompanied by chronic intestinal disorders. Thorough chewing of food is therefore essential, preferably 80 to 100 times or more per mouthful, until the food becomes completely liquified.

6.    It is important for persons with arthritis to have regular, daily bowel movements. If they experience constipation, dishes such as kanten, boiled salad, steamed greens, or vegetables sautéed in a small amount of sesame oil can be eaten. If constipation persists, a mild salt-water or salt-bancha enema can be given.

7.    A hot body scrub using a medium-sized towel dipped in plain, hot water can be done twice per day. Begin with the hands and fingers, and work your way to the arms, shoulders, neck and head, back, abdomen, buttocks, and so on, finishing with the feet and toes. Reheat the towel before you do each section of the body, and scrub until the skin becomes slightly red or the circulation becomes active.
   Part of the problem of arthritis is due to accumulation of excess fat—mostly from animal sources and simple sugars—and minerals in and around the joints. These accumulations are accelerated when a thin layer of fat builds up under the skin, again, due largely to the chronic overconsumption of animal fats. The excessive factors normally discharged through the skin are thus blocked and held within the body. Daily scrubbing helps activate circulation and break these accumulations down.

8.    In severe cases, where the person is experiencing tightness or inflexibility, you may scrub the body with a hot ginger towel instead of using plain hot water. This may be done daily for some period in more severe cases or several times per week in less severe cases.

9.    Hot towel compresses may be applied daily to joints or hardened body parts to relieve pain and dissolve stagnation, except in cases of active inflammation or swelling. Hot ginger towels (ginger compresses) may be used in more severe cases. It is also helpful in more severe cases to soak swollen fingers and hands, or both feet in hot ginger water for about ten minutes.

10.    Another helpful external treatment for arthritic persons is the periodic application of a ginger compress on the abdominal area.

This can be done several times per week or more often in severe cases. Of course, as with all dietary and home applications, it is recommended that advice be sought from a qualified macrobiotic advisor or center.

A further recommendation is to rub down along the spine with a towel dipped in hot ginger water. (This can be especially helpful in cases of ankylosing spondylitis). Soak a towel in the water, squeeze, and then rub the area until it becomes red.

Below are general recommendations for the five major types of arthritis, based on the understanding of their yin or yang causes. For more yang types of arthritis—osteoarthritis, ankylosing spondylitis, and gout—slightly more yin energies are emphasized in the selection and preparation of daily foods. For more yin forms of arthritis, including conditions such as rheumatoid arthritis and lupus, slightly more yang energies are emphasized It bears repeating, though, that all conditions still need both energies, and it is important not to be one-sided in your cooking and selection of foods.

In Chapter 6, guidelines are presented for preparing some of the special dishes and home cares introduced in this section.

## Dietary Recommendations for the Major Types of Arthritis

In the following section, the major types of arthritis are listed with appropriate dietary suggestions. These guidelines provide readers with a dietary outline they can use to help their recovery of health. The effectiveness of these suggestions, that is, how much we can change arthritis, is based on the individual's skill in cooking the recommended foods, and on practices such as chewing thoroughly.

In order to maximize one's opportunity for recovery, it is recommended that the companion cookbook on arthritis in the *Macrobiotic Food and Cooking Series* be consulted. This book contains clear, simple explanations that include the proper selection of foods, easy to follow liefestyle guidelines, and the macrobiotic view of the cause of arthritis.

In addition, we recommend that all persons seeking to implement macrobiotic dietary guidelines contact a macrobiotic center for advice. The guidelines presented below, for example, can be generally observed for several months, at which time adjustments may be required. Also, these guidelines are not substitutes for medical advice. Persons with serious conditions are advised to contact the appropriate medical or nutritional professional in addition to macrobiotic practice.

64

## Dietary Suggestions for Rheumatoid Arthritis

*Whole Grains:*
- Short grain brown rice can be eaten daily, so that it becomes the primary grain. It can be cooked with a pinch of sea salt or a one-half-inch piece of kombu sea vegetable per cup of rice. Brown rice can also be eaten in combination with other grains and smaller types of beans.
- Secondary grains can include millet, whole wheat berries, barley, and others.
- Whole wheat noodles, called *udon*, can be eaten several times per week in soup.
- It is best for the time being to avoid frequent intake of baked flour products such as cookies, crackers, chips, and the like, although high-quality unyeasted sourdough bread can be eaten several times per week.
- Breakfast porridge can be made by adding water to leftover whole grains and cooking them for a short time. This may be eaten daily. Soft brown rice (*kayu*) is an ideal breakfast cereal. Oatmeal made from rolled or steel-cut oats is best avoided temporarily. Cooked whole oats are best.

*Soups:*
- One cup or bowl of miso soup can be taken daily, preferably using either *mugi* (barley) or *Hatcho* (soybean) miso. This soup can include sea vegetables, either wakame or kombu, and a variety of vegetables, especially daikon, leafy greens, and sweet-tasting vegetables. A mild-tasting soup is preferable for daily use.
- A second cup or bowl of soup composed of different ingredients such as whole grains or beans may be taken for variety during the course of the day. It is important to use sea vegetables when preparing soups.

*Vegetables:*
- All three types of vegetables—leafy, round, and root—can be consumed daily, using a variety of cooking styles. However, daikon roots and leaves are especially helpful for this condition and should be included on a regular basis.
- For the first month it is best not to use oil in cooking. During the second month, oil can be used in sautéing about once per week, and during the third month, about twice per week.
- Raw salads are best not taken until the symptoms of arthritis diminish somewhat; however boiled and pressed salads can be eaten daily or every other day.

- *Kinpira* (burdock and carrot dish) and *nishime* style vegetables are helpful for this condition and can be eaten several times per week.
- Contracted leafy greens (daikon, turnip, carrot, etc.) are also helpful.

*Beans and Bean Products:*
- Smaller beans (azuki, chick-pea, lentil, and black soybeans) can be taken daily, about one-half-cup serving size.
- Larger beans are best not eaten for the first month; during the second month they can be taken two or three times per month.
- *Tempeh* and dried tofu can be eaten every other day in a variety of dishes.
- Fresh tofu can be used in small amounts once or twice per week.

*Sea Vegetables:*
- Wakame and kombu are used daily in soup, with vegetables, and with beans.
- Arame and hijiki side dishes can be eaten two three times per week, and a sheet of toasted nori can be consumed daily.
- Sea vegetables can be used daily in moderate amounts.

*Condiments:*
- Condiments such as gomashio and sea vegetable powders can be used in small volume on a daily basis. Gomashio can be made in a 16 to 1 proportion of sesame seeds to sea salt.
- Umeboshi plums can be eaten two or three times per week.
- Roasted shiso leaves and nori condiment are helpful supplementary condiments, and can be eaten two to three times per week, as can tekka.
- It is best to avoid umeboshi or brown rice vinegar during episodes of joint pain.

*Pickles:*
- A small volume of naturally fermented pickles or sauerkraut can be eaten each day.
- Pickles with a strong sour taste are best minimized until the arthritis improves.
- If pickles have an excessively salty flavor, rinse them off briefly under cold water before eating.
- Pickled daikon, known as *takuan* can be helpful when eaten several times per week. Several small slices at a time are enough.

*Fish and Seafood:*
- It is best to use white-meat fish only, about once or twice per week

if desired. Fish can be steamed, broiled, or cooked in soup.
- Fish and seafood are best eaten with a garnish of grated raw daikon or carrot.

*Fruits:*
- With swelling and inflammation, raw fruit or juice is best mini-mized.
- A small, dessert-sized portion of cooked northern varieties of fruit can be eaten several times per week if desired.
- Dried fruit such as raisins or apples can occasionally be used in small amounts for sweetness.
- Among northern fruits, cooked or dried peaches are especially helpful and can be used most often. A small volume of fresh peaches can occasionally be eaten in summer, with a pinch of sea salt.

*Nuts:*
- It is best to limit the intake of nuts and nut butters until the condition improves.
- Dried chestnuts can occasionally be cooked with rice, sweet rice, or azuki beans for a sweet flavor.

*Seeds:*
- A small volume of lightly roasted sesame, pumpkin, or squash seeds can be eaten.
- Sunflower seeds are best avoided temporarily or taken only in summertime in small volume.

*Snacks:*
- A moderate amount of snacks such as popcorn, rice cakes, and puffed cereals can be eaten.
- Sushi, rice balls, leftovers, noodles, and occasional sourdough bread can also be eaten in moderate amounts as snacks.

*Sweet Vegetables:*
- Several varieties of sweet vegetables such as carrots, squash, onions, and cabbage can be used daily in cooking.

*Additional Sweets:*
- Brown rice syrup is the preferred concentrated grain sweetener for this condition. Several teaspoons per week can be added to break-fast cereal, tea, or used in making dessert.

*Beverages:*
- Beverages such as bancha tea, spring water, and grain teas may be consumed as thirst requires. Other suggested beverages can be taken on an occasional basis.
- A half cup of carrot juice, not icy cold, may be taken once or twice per week. However, if there is pain in the joints, it is best to wait before including it.

*Seasoning:*
- Miso, tamari soy sauce, sea salt, and other seasonings are best used moderately in cooking.
- Seasonings that are more stimulating, such as ginger and horse-radish, are best minimized for the time being.

*Special Drinks.*
- Sweet vegetable broth can be taken, one cup daily.
- *Ume-sho-kuzu* can be taken twice per week for several weeks.
- Grated daikon (1/3 of a cup) plus grated carrot (1/3 of a cup) with water added to make one full cup can also be included several times per week for one month. These ingredients are simmered for two to three minutes with a few drops of tamari soy sauce.
- Roasted brown rice tea can be used alternately with bancha as a primary beverage for this condition.

*Home Care:*
- For swollen, hot joints, a plaster made of raw leafy greens mashed in a suribachi, or a tofu and greens plaster (mash equal proportions together in a suribachi) can be applied directly to the painful joint.

*Lifestyle Suggestions*
- Use a hot, damp cloth to scrub the body daily, morning and evening before bed.
- Chew very well, until food turns into liquid.
- Do not take extra-long baths or showers.
- Rings, watches, and other jewelry and metallic accessories are best not worn, especially in areas where the joint is painful.

## Dietary Suggestions for Lupus

*Whole Grains:*
- Pressure-cooked short grain brown rice can be eaten daily, by itself or in combination with other grains and smaller beans.
- Secondary grains such as barley, millet, and corn on the cob (when in season) can be prepared.

- Whole wheat noodles, called udon, can be eaten several times per week in broth.
- It is best for a time to avoid baked flour products, except for occasional sourdough, unyeasted bread.
- Buckwheat noodles, called soba, and whole grain buckwheat, called kasha, can be eaten once per week or so to help strengthen the condition; however, not if skin disease is being experienced.

*Soups:*
- One cup or bowl of miso soup can be taken daily, seasoned with the proper amount of mugi or Hatcho miso. Wakame or kombu, plus a good variety of vegetables, can also be used.
- A second cup or bowl of soup that includes a different combination of ingredients and seasonings can be enjoyed every day for variety.

*Vegetables:*
- A wide variety of vegetables can be eaten daily, using the full range of cooking styles. Burdock root is especially helpful for this condition and can be included several times per week.
  Raw salad is best avoided for a while, so boiled and pressed salads, or steamed greens, can be used daily.
- The use of oil in cooking can be avoided for about one month. During the second month, oil can be used once per week; during the third month, once or twice per week.
- Among special dishes, azuki beans cooked with squash and kombu; burdock and carrot kinpira; daikon, carrots, and turnips, cooked with their green tops; dried, shredded daikon cooked with kombu; and nishime are especially helpful.

*Beans and Bean Products:*
- Smaller, low-fat beans (azuki, chick-pea, lentil, black soybean) are preferred for daily use. The volume consumed can be up to one-half cup per day.
- The larger, more fatty beans are best avoided for the first month. After this, they can be included once every 10 days or so.
- Bean products like tempeh, tofu, and dried tofu can be included three or four times per week.

*Sea Vegetables:*
- Kombu and wakame can be used daily in soups, with vegetables, and in bean or other dishes.
- Hijiki or arame can be made in separate side dishes and included two or three times per week.

- A sheet of toasted nori can be consumed daily with rice balls or
  or sushi, or as a garnish or snack.

*Condiments:*
  Gomashio and sea-vegetable powders can be used daily. Gomashio
  can be made in a 16 to 1 proportion of sesame seeds to sea salt.
  High-quality black sesame seeds are helpful if the can be obtained.
- Umeboshi plums can be used three or four times per week with
  whole grains or with tea.
- Two special condiments can be used several times per week: shio
  kombu and nori condiments. (Use one or two pieces of shio kombu
  or a teaspoon of nori condiment at a time.)
- In cases of inflammation, it is best to minimize or avoid the use of
  brown rice vinegar and umeboshi vinegar until the condition
  improves.
- Tekka, a special condiment made from carrot, burdock, lotus root,
  and miso can be helpful when eaten with brown rice or other grains
  two or three times per week in small amounts.

*Pickles:*
- A daily, small volume of pickles can be taken after meals.
- If the taste is excessively salty, pickles can be briefly rinsed off
  under cold water before eating.
- It is best to minimize or avoid very salty or very sour pickles.

*Fish and Seafood:*
- A small portion of white-meat fish can be prepared once or twice
  per week if necessary.
- If someone with lupus begins to feel very weak and lacks vitality,
  then carp soup (*Koi-koku*) can be taken for several days (one cup
  or bowl per day), and again one or two weeks later.

*Fruits:*
- If craved, a half cup of cooked northern fruit (with a pinch of sea
  salt) can be eaten several times per week.
- Raw fruits are best avoided until the condition improves.
- Dried chestnuts, when cooked with brown rice, sweet brown rice,
  or azuki beans are preferred over fruit. They can be eaten several
  times per week if desired.

*Nuts:*
- It is best not to eat nuts or nut butters until the condition improves
  and then only occasionally in small volume as snacks.

*Seeds:*
- A small volume of lightly roasted sesame, pumpkin, or squash seeds can be eaten as snacks.
  Sunflower seeds are best avoided until summer, and then eaten only on occasion in small quantities.

*Snacks:*
- Be careful not to eat too many dry snacks, such as rice cakes, popcorn, or puffed cereals, as these can cause a craving for liquid or sweets.
- Other snacks can be consumed moderately.

*Sweet Vegetables:*
- Sweet-tasting vegetables such as onions, squash, carrots, and cabbage can be used daily in cooking.

*Additional Sweets:*
- Minimize the use of concentrated sweeteners such as rice syrup or barley malt. If strongly craved, a small volume can be taken several times per week.
- Among concentrated natural sweeteners, the carbohydrate, or sugar, found in carrots can be especially helpful. Carrots can be simmered for a long time over a low flame to make carrot butter or carrot concentrate. Carrot butter can be used several times per week as a spread (on rice cakes or sourdough bread) or as a sweet condiment. Carrot concentrate can be dissolved in water and taken as a drink several times per week.

*Beverages:*
- Beverages such as bancha twig tea, grain teas, or grain coffee can be taken according to need.
- Carrot juice (about 1/2 cup) can be enjoyed several times per week, and if symptoms are active, can be added later.

*Seasonings:*
- Seasonings are best used moderately.
- Seasonings that are more stimulating, such as ginger and horse-radish, are best avoided until the condition improves.

*Special Drinks:*
- Sweet vegetable broth can be taken, about one cup daily.
- Ume-sho-kuzu can be taken twice per week for about three weeks.

*Home Care:*
- A hot ginger compress or repeated hot towels (for 10 to 15 minutes) can be applied to the kidneys (middle back) and intestines (lower abdomen) to strengthen these organs in their functions of eliminating excess. These compresses can be done about two or three times per week for about six weeks.

*Lifestyle Suggestions:*
- It is important to chew very well, until food becomes liquid in the mouth.
- Every morning and evening before bed, a complete body scrub can be done with a cotton towel that is held under the hot faucet and wrung out.
- A half-hour daily walk is suggested as a comfortable form of exercise.
- Do not take long hot baths or showers.
- As much as possible try to obtain quality organic grains, beans, and vegetables.

**Dietary Suggestions for Osteoarthritis**

*Whole Grains:*
- Short grain brown rice can be pressure-cooked with a pinch of sea salt and eaten daily. Brown rice can also be cooked in combination with other grains and smaller beans.
- Barley, especially pearl barley (*hato mugi*), can also be helpful. It can be eaten two or three times per week with rice or in the form of soup.
- Secondary grains such as barley, millet, and corn on the cob (when in season) can be used.
- It is best to limit the intake of baked flour products. If bread is craved, natural-quality sourdough (unyeasted) can be eaten several times per week, preferably steamed until soft.
- It is best to avoid rolled or steel-cut oats, as well as other cracked or flaked grains until improvement occurs. If oats are craved, cook whole oats overnight on a very low flame.
- Noodles, preferably whole wheat noodles, called udon, can be eaten several times a week in broth.

*Soup:*
- Soups are best when seasoned very lightly, avoiding a strong salty taste.
- One cup or bowl of miso soup can be taken daily with wakame,

72

kombu, and a variety of vegetables, especially daikon, shiitake mushroom, and leafy greens.
- Miso soup can be garnished with chopped scallions, chives, or parsley.
- A variety of other soups can be used each day as a second cup or bowl.

*Vegetables:*
- A wide range of vegetables can be eaten daily using a variety of combinations and cooking styles.
- Cooked dandelions are especially helpful and can be included two or three times per week when available.
- Raw salad is best avoided until the condition improves; however, the energy of boiled salad and steamed greens can be helpful, and these dishes can be included daily. Occasional raw salad can be added once the condition improves.
- The use of oil in cooking is best avoided for one month. During the second month, a small amount of sesame oil can be used several times per week.

*Beans and Bean Products:*
- Smaller beans (azuki, chick-pea, lentil, and black soybean) are preferable for daily use.
- Bean products can be eaten daily or every other day.
- If someone is overweight, it is best to avoid larger beans for one month, after which they can be included once every week or 10 days.

*Sea Vegetables:*
- Kombu and wakame can be taken daily in soup, vegetables, and in bean dishes.
- Hijiki or arame can be prepared as side dishes two or three times per week.
- A sheet of toasted nori can be eaten daily.

*Condiments:*
- Gomashio and sea vegetable powders can be used daily. Gomashio can be made in a 16 to 1 proportion of sesame seeds to sea salt.
- Umeboshi plums can be eaten two or three times per week, as can a small volume of brown rice or umeboshi vinegar.

*Pickles:*
- A small volume of pickles may be eaten daily. If the taste is

excessively salty, they can be briefly washed in cold water before eating.
- Quick, light pickles or sauerkraut are preferred for more regular use.

*Fish and Seafood:*
- A small portion of white-meat fish can be eaten once or twice per week if desired.
- Shellfish and more fatty fish (e.g., tuna, salmon, etc.) are best minimized or avoided until the condition improves.
- Fish can be prepared by either boiling, steaming, or in miso soup.

*Fruit:*
- Cooked northern fruits can be enjoyed as dessert about three times per week.
- Plums are especially helpful and can be cooked in dessert from time to time.
- Raw fruit is best kept to a minimum until the condition improves.

*Nuts:*
- It is best to avoid nuts or nut butters until the condition improves, at which time they can be included from time to time in snacks.

*Seeds:*
- A small volume of lightly roasted sesame, pumpkin, or squash seeds can be eaten as snacks. Do not burn the seeds while roasting.
- Sunflower seeds are best avoided until summer, at which time they can be eaten in small quantities on occasion.

*Snacks:*
- Be careful not to eat too many dry snacks, such as rice cakes, popcorn, and puffed cereals.
- Other snacks can be consumed according to desire.

*Sweet Vegetables:*
- These can be used daily in cooking.

*Additional Sweets:*
- A small volume of barley malt (about one teaspoon) can be used several times per week on breakfast porridge, in dessert, or in tea.
- Other concentrated sweeteners can be used occasionally.
- Dried chestnuts may be cooked with brown rice or azuki beans from time to time as a sweet treat.

*Beverages:*
- Bancha twig tea, spring water, and grain teas can be taken daily. The volume depends on how thirsty a person is.
- Roasted barley tea (*mugicha*) or pearl barley tea (*hato mugicha*) are especially helpful and can be alternated with bancha as main beverages.

*Seasonings:*
- Seasonings are best used moderately in daily cooking.
- Seasonings that are more stimulating, such as ginger and horse-radish, are best avoided until the condition improves.

*Special Drinks:*
- Sweet vegetable broth can be taken, about one cup daily for one month or longer if necessary.
- A drink made from fresh grated daikon (1/3 of a cup), grated carrot (1/3 of a cup), and 1/3 cup of water can be taken two or three times per week for one month. Simmer for two or three minutes with a few drops of tamari soy sauce.
- Dandelion coffee, available at most natural food stores, is especially helpful for this condition. It can be used three or four times per week as a supplement to other beverages.

*Home Care:*
- Hot towels or a hot ginger compress can be applied to painful joints whenever necessary to improve circulation and reduce hardening.

*Lifestyle Suggestions:*
- It is important to chew very well, until food becomes liquid in the mouth.
- Every morning and evening before bed, a complete body scrub can be done with a hot cotton towel.
- A half-hour daily walk is suggested as a form of comfortable exercise.
- A short shower or bath can be taken daily.

**Dietary Suggestions for Ankylosing Spondylitis**

*Whole Grains:*
- Short grain brown rice can be used daily, with medium grain used occasionally as a supplement. Brown rice can also be cooked in combination with other grains and beans.

- It is best not to cook grains until they become dry, so a little extra water can be used.
- Among the secondary grains, fresh corn and barley can be helpful.
- Corn on the cob can be eaten often when it is available.
- It is best for a time to minimize or avoid flour products such as cookies, crackers, muffins, and the like. Unyeasted sourdough bread—preferably steamed until soft—can be eaten several times per week.
- If oats are craved, whole oats can be cooked overnight over a very low flame and eaten for breakfast.
- Whole wheat udon can be eaten several times a week in light tamari broth.
- Buckwheat noodles and whole grain buckwheat are best avoided until the condition improves.
- Naturally processed corn grits can be used several times per week as a breakfast cereal.

*Soup:*
- One cup or bowl of miso soup, with wakame or kombu, and a variety of vegetables, can be included daily. Summer greens, daikon, and shiitake mushrooms can be included in miso soup.
- A second bowl or cup of soup may be included daily using a variety of other ingredients and seasonings. Corn and vegetable soup can be included several times per week.
- It is important to use a small piece of sea vegetable in preparing soup.

*Vegetables:*
- All three types of vegetables—leafy, root, and round—can be eaten daily using a variety of combinations and cooking styles.
- Among acceptable vegetables, cucumber is helpful to relax an overly tight condition. It can be served several times per week in salad and used to make pickles.
- The use of sesame oil in cooking is best kept to several times per week.
- Boiled salad and quickly steamed greens can be helpful when included daily.

*Beans and Bean Products:*
- The smaller beans (azuki, chick-pea, lentil, and black soybean) and bean products can be used alternately on a daily basis. The volume consumed can average about one-half cup daily.
- The larger beans are best taken about two to three times per month.

*Sea Vegetables:*
- Kombu and wakame can be eaten daily in soup, with vegetables, and in bean dishes.
- Hijiki or arame can be cooked as side dishes two or three times per week.
- A sheet of toasted nori can be eaten daily with rice-balls, sushi, or as a garnish.

*Condiments:*
- Gomashio and sea-vegetable powders can be used daily. Gomashio can be made in a 16 to 1 proportion of sesame seeds to sea salt.
- Umeboshi plums can be eaten two or three times per week.
- It is best to minimize the use of brown rice vinegar and umeboshi vinegar if there is pain.
- Other condiments may be used several times per week.

*Pickles:*
- A small volume of pickles may be eaten daily. Quick, light pickles, including natural, non-spicy cucumber pickles, are preferred.
- If the taste is excessively salty, they can be briefly washed in cold water before eating.

*Fish and Seafood:*
- A small portion of white-meat fish can be eaten once or twice per week.
- Other varieties of fish or shellfish are best avoided until the condition improves.

*Fruit:*
- Among fruits, apricots can be helpful for this condition. They, along with other cooked northern fruits, can be enjoyed about three times per week on average. A small volume of dried apricots can be eaten on occasion, as can a small amount of fresh apricots in season.

*Nuts:*
- It is best to minimize or avoid nuts or nut butters until the condition improves.

*Seeds:*
- A small volume of lightly roasted sesame, pumpkin, or squash seeds can be eaten as snacks. It is important not to take a large amount of dry, roasted seeds.

- Sunflower seeds are best avoided until summer and then can be eaten in small quantities.

*Snacks:*
- A reduced volume of dry snacks such as rice cakes, popcorn, and puffed cereals is best. However, puffed whole corn can be helpful and can be used as a frequent snack. It can be eaten plain or together with amazaké.
- Other snacks can be consumed moderately.

*Sweet Vegetables:*
- These can be used in daily cooking.

*Additional Sweets:*
- If extra sweetness is craved, a small volume of rice syrup, barley malt, or amasaké can be included several times per week.
- Corn amazaké can be especially helpful in this case.
- Dried chestnuts may also be cooked with grains or beans for added sweetness.

*Beverages:*
- Bancha tea, spring water, and grain teas can be taken daily. The amount depends upon how thirsty an individual is.
- Carrot or apricot juice can be used once or twice per week if desired.
- All drinks should be warm or room temperature.

*Seasonings:*
- Seasonings are best used moderately in daily cooking.
- Seasonings that are more stimulating, such as ginger and horse-radish, are best avoided for the time being.

*Special Drinks:*
- Sweet vegetable broth can be taken two or three times per week.
- Grated carrot (1/3 of a cup) plus grated daikon (1/3 of a cup) can be taken several times per week, either raw or simmered. A few drops of tamari soy sauce can be added.

*Home Care:*
- Hot towels or a hot ginger compress can be applied to painful areas of the spine, especially when symptoms are present.
- The whole spine can also be rubbed vigorously with either of the above hot compresses.

*Lifestyle Suggestions:*
- It is important to chew really well, until food becomes liquid in the mouth.
- Every morning and evening before bed, a complete body scrub can be done with a hot cotton cloth.
- A daily short shower or bath can be taken.
- If possible, a half-hour walk is suggested as a comfortable form of exercise.
- Do not let yourself become cold which can cause tightness.

*Special Suggestions:*
- It is important to use sea salt, miso, and other seasonings in a moderate, balanced way so that food does not have an overly salty flavor.

## Dietary Suggestions for Gout

*Whole Grains*
- Short grain brown rice can be the main grain for daily use. It can be cooked with other grains and with azuki and other beans.
- Millet can be featured as a secondary grain, along with barley, fresh corn, and others.
- It is best for a time to avoid baked flour products such as cookies, muffins, and crackers, even those of natural, organic quality, until the condition improves.
- High-quality, sourdough bread can be eaten several times per week.
- If oats are craved, whole oats can be used as breakfast cereal.
- Whole wheat noodles, called udon, can be eaten several times a week in broth, while buckwheat is best avoided until the condition improves.
- Creamy, floury cereals or sauces are also best avoided.

*Soup:*
- One cup or bowl of miso soup can be included daily with wakame or kombu and a variety of vegetables, especially daikon, shiitake mushroom, and leafy greens.
- A variety of other soups can be included, including millet and squash soup, pureed squash soup, and azuki bean soup.

*Vegetables:*
- Leafy, green, round, and root vegetables can be eaten daily, using a variety of combinations and cooking styles.
- Cabbage is especially helpful for this condition and can be served

often, as can other sweet vegetables such as squash and onions.

- Raw salad is best minimized or avoided until the condition improves.
- The use of oil is best kept to a minimum. If swelling and pain are experienced, it may be necessary to avoid oil temporarily.
- Squash cooked with azuki beans and kombu can be helpful in providing additional sweetness and can be included two or four times per week.

*Beans and Bean Products:*
- Smaller beans (azuki, chick-peas, lentil, and black soybean) can be used daily. The volume consumed can average about one-half cup.
- Tempeh, tofu, dried tofu, and natto can also be included three or four times per week.
- If someone is overweight, it is best to avoid larger, fattier beans for about a month. Afterward, they can be used weekly.

*Sea Vegetables:*
- Kombu and wakame can be used daily in soups, with vegetables, and in bean dishes.
- Hijiki or arame can be included in side dishes two or three times per week.
- A sheet of toasted nori can be eaten daily.

*Condiments:*
- Gomashio and sea-vegetable powders can be used daily. Gomashio can be made in a 16 to 1 proportion of sesame seeds to sea salt.
- Umeboshi plums can be eaten two or three times per week.
- Other condiments may be used several times per week for variety.
- It is best to minimize the use of brown rice and umeboshi vinegar, especially when there is joint pain.

*Pickles:*
- A small volume of pickles can be eaten daily. If the taste is excessively salty, they can be briefly washed in cold water before eating.

*Fish and Seafood:*
- Excessive consumption of animal protein and fat contributes to this condition. Therefore, it is best to eat a small proportion of white-meat fish only once or twice per week if craved. Fish can be eaten along with several tablespoons of grated raw daikon as garnish.
- Other varieties of seafood are best avoided until the condition improves.

*Fruit:*
- Cooked northern fruit can be eaten about three times a week as a dessert.
- Raw or dried fruits can be eaten occasionally in small volume if desired.

*Sweet Vegetables:*
- These can be used daily in cooking.

*Additional Sweets:*
- A small volume of concentrated sweeteners can be used once or twice a week if desired.
- Amazaké can also be used on occasion.

*Beverages:*
- Bancha tea, spring water, and grain teas can be used daily.
- Carrot juice can be enjoyed several times per week if desired.
- It is important to avoid icy cold beverages and to not drink excessively.

*Seasonings:*
- Seasonings are best used moderately. Seasonings that are more stimulating, such as ginger or horseradish, are best avoided until the condition improves.

*Special Drinks:*
- Sweet vegetable broth can be included two or three times per week, a cup at a time.
- Grated carrot (1/3 of a cup), grated daikon (1/3 of a cup), and water can be taken two to three times per week for one month. Simmer this mixture over a low flame for two or three minutes and add tamari soy sauce.
- Kombu tea can also be taken several times per week until the condition improves.

*Home Care:*
- For pain in the joints, a tofu and raw greens plaster (half and half mashed in a suribachi) can be applied directly to the painful area.
- Raw greens or tofu can also be applied separately. These can be applied when the joint is painful, or two to three times per week for a month.
- A hot ginger compress can be applied to the kidney region twice a week for one month.

*Lifestyle Suggestions:*
- It is important to chew very well, until the food becomes liquid in the mouth.
- Every morning and evening before bed, a complete body scrub can be done with a hot cotton towel.
- A half-hour daily walk is suggested as a comfortable form of exercise.
- A daily short shower or bath can be taken.
- It is best not to smoke.
- If the large-toe area is afflicted—which happens in most cases of gout—it is important to wear cotton socks.

# 6. Arthritis Home Care ━━━━━━━━

As we saw in Chapter 3, arthritis develops as the result of chronic accumulation of excess in and around the joints. Various conditions of discharge and accumulation often precede degeneration of the bones, joints, and connective tissues. Common symptoms, such as digestive upsets, colds, fever, diarrhea, acne, and others indicate that the body is attempting to discharge excess, the root cause of which is imbalance in the daily diet.

In the macrobiotic view, symptoms such as these can be beneficial. They help the body to discharge execess and thereby remain free of arthritis and other serious illnesses. When we are generally eating well, minor problems can usually be managed at home by changing one's way of eating (especially by avoiding the foods that are producing imbalance), preparing a variety of special dishes, and with simple home care.

Below are a variety of natural preparations that can be made at home in the kitchen. They can help in the relief of minor problems such as colds, coughing, skin discharges, fever, and digestive upsets. When properly applied, traditional home remedies are completely safe and do not produce undesirable side effects. They have been used as a part of natural lifestyles for thousands of years.

The special drinks and other forms of home care listed below are presented for educational purposes and are not substitutes for qualified medical advice. Anyone with arthritis or another serious condition is advised to seek the appropriate medical advice. Moreover, do not hesitate to contact a qualified macrobiotic teacher or center for guidance on the proper use of these natural home cares.

For further information on using many of the food items presented in this section, please see the companion cookbook in the *Macrobiotic Food and Cooking Series* titled, *Arthritis*, by Aveline Kushi, edited by Wendy Esko. This book offers a variety of recipes, menus, and ideas for meal planning according to macrobiotic principles.

## Drinks and Garnishes ━━━━━━━━━━

### Azuki Bean Tea

Azuki beans are small and compact in size, oblong in shape, and red or brown in color. They contain less fat and oil than other beans, and in the Far East where they originated are considered an honorary grain. They are enjoyed as a small side dish, in soup, cooked with grains, and in desserts. They have become a staple in many macrobiotic and natural food diets.

Tea made from high-grade azuki beans (which have a deep maroon color and a shiny surface) can be used to soften hard stools and strengthen the kidneys. The intestines and kidneys are major organs of discharge. It is important that they function properly in order to keep the body free of toxic accumulations that can lead to arthritis.

*To prepare:* Place 1 cup of washed azuki beans in a pot. Add 3 to 4 cups of water, and a strip of kombu about an inch long. Bring to boil, cover, and reduce the flame to low. Simmer 30 to 45 minutes. Strain out the liquid.

Azuki bean tea can be included along with other beverages for several days or longer. The leftover beans can be used in soups or cooked with rice.

## Bancha Twig Tea

Bancha tea is picked in midsummer from the large and mature leaves, stems, and twigs of the tea bush. These are called respectively bancha leaf tea, bancha stem tea, and bancha twig tea. Traditionally picked by hand in the high mountains, the bancha leaves, stems, and twigs are roasted and cooled up to four separate times in large iron cauldrons. This procedure, as well as the late harvest when the caffeine has naturally receded from the tea bush, makes for a tea containing virtually no caffeine or tannin, especially in the stem and twig parts.

Also, unlike other teas which are acidic, bancha is slightly alkaline and thus has a soothing, beneficial effect on digestion, blood quality, and the mind. It is entirely safe for even infants and small children to drink. In most macrobiotic households, bancha is the most commonly consumed beverage, usually served after every meal and in-between meals.

Bancha twig tea is also known as *kukicha* tea, from the Japanese words for "twig tea."

*To prepare:* Place a tablespoon of twigs in a quart of water and bring to boil. Reduce the flame to low and simmer for 3 to 5 minutes (for a mild tea) or 10 to 15 minutes (for a stronger beverage).

## Daikon Tea 1

Daikon, or white radish, is an indispensable part of traditional Far

Eastern cuisine and is now grown in America. The smaller, thinner daikon, shaped somewhat like a carrot, grows more quickly than the larger varieties and has a strong, sharp taste. The big juicy ones grow up to several feet in length and are sweeter to the taste.

Tea made from grated raw daikon was traditionally used to help reduce fever by inducing sweating. (It is not recommended for someone with a weakened condition or for small children.)

*To prepare:* Grate 1 to 2 tablespoons of daikon radish, and place in a tea cup. Add 1/4 to 1/2 teaspoon of fresh grated ginger, and a tablespoon of tamari soy sauce. Pour weak, hot bancha tea or boiling water over the ingredients. Stir and drink hot.

## Daikon Tea 2

This variation of daikon tea can be used to induce urination and calm and relax the body.

*To prepare:* Grate a small amount of daikon, and place it in a piece of cheesecloth. Squeeze 2 tablespoons of juice through the cloth and mix it with about 6 tablespoons of water. Place in a saucepan and add a pinch of sea salt. Bring to a boil, reduce the flame to low, and simmer for about a minute. Drink hot.

Take only once per day. It is better not to use this drink for more than 3 days in a row unless otherwise indicated.

## Daikon Tea 3

This drink helps dissolve deposits of fat and mucus in the body, especially those resulting from overconsumption of fats and oils.

Place 1 tablespoon of fresh grated daikon in a tea cup. Add 1 teaspoon of tamari soy sauce, and pour hot bancha tea over the mixture. Drink hot.

As with the other daikon teas, it is usually better not to use this drink for more than 2 or 3 days unless otherwise indicated.

## Daikon-Carrot Drink

Grated daikon and carrot can be used to help the body discharge fats and dissolve hardened accumulations in the intestinal tract and in the joints.

Grate 1 tablespoon each of fresh daikon and carrot. Place 2 cups of water in a saucepan. Add the daikon and carrot and a pinch of sea salt. Bring to boil, reduce the flame to low, and simmer for 5 to 8 minutes.

**Dried Daikon Tea**

This drink can be used to help reduce fever in a person who is unable
to use raw grated daikon.

*To prepare:* Place 1/4 cup of dried daikon in a saucepan and add
2 cups of water. Bring to a boil, reduce the flame to low, and cover.
Simmer for about 10 minutes. Drink while hot.

**Grated Daikon Garnish**

Grated raw daikon can alo be used as a garnish to help digest oily or
fatty foods, such as *tempura* or mochi, and to help the body meta-
olize the oils and fats in fish and other animal foods.

*To prepare:* Grate 1 to 2 tablespoons of fresh, uncooked daikon
and sprinkle several drops of tamari soy sauce over it. You may
also add a dab of fresh grated ginger for a slightly stronger garnish.
Place several tablespoons on the plate along with the foods mentioned above, and eat along with them.

**Fresh Lotus Root Tea**

In Far Eastern countries, lotus root has been known for centuries as
being effective in easing respiratory problems, including coughs and
congestion. The root of the lotus flower plant grows underwater in
segmented lengths, is light brown in color, and contains hollow cham-
bers. It can be regularly included in a variety of dishes—such as with
other root vegetables or with sea vegetables—or can be used to
prepare tea or external plasters.

*To prepare lotus root tea:* Wash and then grate a 4-inch piece of
lotus root. Place in a piece of cheesecloth and squeeze all of the
liquid into a measuring cup. Add an equal amount of water to the
the lotus juice and place in a saucepan. Add a small pinch of sea
salt and bring to a boil. Reduce the flame to low and simmer for
3 to 5 minutes. Drink 1 to 2 cups per day for several days.

**Powdered Lotus Root Tea**

Pre-packaged, powdered lotus root tea is available in most natural
and macrobiotic food stores. It can be used when fresh lotus root is
not available. Directions for making it are printed on the package.
Tea made from powdered lotus root can be used in the same manner
as tea made from fresh lotus root.

### Kombu Tea

Kombu, a brown algae, belongs to the *Laminaria* family of sea vegetables which includes some kelps, oarweed, tangle, and other deep-sea varieties. The color of Japanese kombu ranges from dark brown to black and the plant has wide, thick fronds. It is gathered off the southern coast of Hokkaido, Japan's northernmost island. Harvested in middle to late summer by boatmen with long poles, kombu is initially wind- and sun-dried and then stored for two to three years in a dark place before being sold in a variety of grades and sizes.

In traditional medicine, sea vegetables have been especially identified with strengthening the heart, the blood, and the circulatory system. They are also excellent for the kidneys, the urinary system, and reproductive organs. They give elasticity to arteries, veins, organ tissues, and joints, contributing to flexibility and the smooth functioning of the body's many interrelated systems.

Like all edible sea vegetables, kombu is rich in essential minerals and other nutrients, and helps the body discharge toxic accumulation in the organs, blood vessels, and joints. Tea made by boiling kombu supplies additional nutrients. There are two basic ways to prepare kombu tea:

1. Place 1 quart of water in a pot and add 1 strip of washed kombu, 3 to 4 inches long. Bring to a boil, cover, and simmer until 2 cups of liquid remain.
2. Place a 6-inch strip of kombu in a 350° F. oven and bake for 10 to 15 minutes or until crisp and brittle but not burnt. Place the roasted kombu in a suribachi and grind to a fine powder. Place 1/2 to 1 teaspoon of the powdered kombu in a cup and pour boiling water over it. Stir and drink while hot.

You can drink a cup of either of these teas for several days in a row, or can enjoy them as a regular beverage several times per week.

### Roasted Barley or Brown Rice Tea

Like bancha, whole grain teas help stabilize overall metabolism. They also help with the gradual elimination of excess coming from overconsumption of animal fats and proteins. These teas are especially helpful in relieving dry skin, especially on the hands and feet, and in strengthening the lungs and large intestine (in the case of brown rice), and the liver and gall bladder (in the case of barley).

*To prepare:* Place 1 to 2 tablespoons of roasted barley or 1/4 cup of dry-roasted brown rice in a quart of water. Bring to a boil, reduce the flame to low, and simmer for about 10 minutes.

Either of these teas can be used daily as one of your staple beverages. Barley tea is especially helpful in offsetting hardening or stiffness in the joints produced by excessive consumption of animal food.

### Shiitake Mushroom Tea

Shiitake mushrooms are originally native to the Far East, and are now grown in America. They are delicious and have been used, fresh or dried, for centuries to balance heavy animal-food intake and for other medicinal purposes. Shiitake tea can be used to relax an overly tight condition in the joints resulting from too much salt or animal food.

*To Prepare:*   Place 1 shiitake in a saucepan. Add 2 cups of water. Bring to a boil, reduce the flame to low, and cover. Simmer together with a small pinch of sea salt or 1 teaspoon of tamari soy sauce until 1 cup of water remains. Strain and drink 1/2 cup at a time while hot.

### Tamari-Bancha Tea

Tamari bancha is easy to make. It promotes circulation and helps neutralize an overly acidic blood condition. It can also help relieve headaches caused by overconsumption of sugar, alcohol, or other acid-producing foods and beverages, and to help restore vitality.

*To prepare:*   Pour 1 to 2 teaspoons of tamari soy sauce into a tea cup. Pour hot bancha tea over it and stir. Drink while hot.

### Tamari-Kuzu

Kuzu (or kudzu as it is known in the southern United States where it is found in abundance) grows wild in the mountains of Japan and has very deep roots. It is traditionally harvested and processed by hand into a white chalklike substance. It is often used in macrobiotic cooking as a thickener in sauces, stews, and desserts. Its medicinal properties include strengthening the digestive organs. Tamari kuzu can be used to fortify digestion, increase vitality, and to relieve fatigue.

*To prepare:*   Place a heaped teaspoon of kuzu powder in a saucepan and add 2 teaspoons of water. Mix until the kuzu is completely dissolved. Add a cup of water and continue mixing. Bring to a boil, reduce the flame to low, and simmer until translucent and thick. Stir constantly to prevent the kuzu from lumping. Add 1/2 to 1 teaspoon of tamari soy sauce and mix. Simmer for another minute, pour into a bowl or cup, and drink while hot.

### Umeboshi Tea

Umeboshi plums grow in the warmer, southern and middle regions of Japan and are related to the apricot. Traditionally fermented with sea salt and pickled with shiso leaves (which give them a deep reddish-purple color), umeboshi have a tangy flavor, combining sour and salty tastes. They are a balanced food, give a strong centering energy, and have a wide range of uses in macrobiotic cooking and home care.

The sourness of the plums draws saliva from the salivary glands, which, when combined with their strong alkalizing effects, helps strengthen the stomach and digestive organs. They can be used to help offset diarrhea, upset stomach and other digestive disorders, and to neutralize an overly acid blood condition.

There are a number of ways to use umboshi in home remedies. *To prepare umeboshi tea:* Bake a plum in the oven until it becomes completely black and crisp. Grind the baked plum in a suribachi until it becomes a fine powder. Place a tablespoon of the powder in a cup and pour hot water over it. Mix well and drink hot.

### Ume-Sho-Bancha

Ume-sho-bancha (umeboshi, plus tamari, plus bancha) helps fortify the blood and activate circulation. It can be used to help relieve fatigue or weakness, and ease a headache, especially when the pain is centered in the front of the head.

*To prepare:* Place 1/2 to 1 plum in a cup with 1/2 to 1 teaspoon of tamari soy sauce. Add hot bancha tea, stir and drink hot.

### Ume-Sho-Bancha with Ginger

Adding a pinch of grated ginger to the above tea makes blood circulation even more active and helps warm the body.

Prepare as above, but add 1/4 teaspoon of freshly grated ginger. Mix well and drink while hot.

### Ume-Sho-Kuzu

This preparation combines the effects of umeboshi and kuzu. It can be used to strengthen the intestines and digestive system as a whole and restore active energy. Ume-sho-kuzu is frequently used to relieve diarrhea or constipation caused by overly weak or expanded intestines. Stagnation in the intestines contributes to the accumulation of toxic excess throughout the body, including hardening, stiffness, or swelling in the joints.

*To prepare:* Dilute a heaped teaspoon of ku·u powder in 2 tea-spoons of water. Add another cup of water ar d mix well. Separate the meat of an umeboshi plum from the seed, and add it. Bring the water to a boil, stirring constantly to prevent lumping. Reduce the flame to low and simmer until thick and translacent. Near the end, add 1/2 to 1 teaspoon of tamari soy sauce and simmer for several more seconds. For a lighter preparation, you can add a small amount of grated ginger at the end. Pour into a bowl or cup and drink hot.

## Condiments

### Gomashio

Gomashio, or "sesame salt," is made from ground, roasted sesame seeds and roasted sea salt. It is the most commonly used macrobiotic condiment, and has a salty-bitter taste that balances the natural sweetness of brown rice and other grains and vegetables.

The proportion of sesame seeds to salt varies from 8 to 1, to 16 to 1 depending on the age and level of activity of each person. For very active adults, the generally recommended ratio of salt to sesame seeds is slightly higher than for ordinary adults, while for less active adults and children, the proportion of salt is lower. Gomashio is delicious, and care must be taken not to overconsume it. A half teaspoon to one teaspoon on a bowl of rice is usually plenty.

Gomashio contains a high amount of calcium, iron, and other nutrients and is an excellent way to obtain polyunsaturated, vegetable-quality oil in whole form. Also, because they are roasted, the sesame seeds in gomashio are easier to digest. The roasted salt with which they are combined provides a harmonious balance to the oil in the seeds. A recipe for gomashio is presented in the companion cook-book, *Arthritis*, by Aveline Kushi, edited by Wendy Esko.

Gomashio can be used to help restore elasticity to the joints and connective tissues. Eating a naturally balanced diet and including foods such as gomashio and sea vegetables is a safe and effective way to restore health and flexibility to the body.

### Shio Kombu

This condiment can help in strengthening the joints and connective tissues.

*To prepare:* Cut 8 twelve-inch strips of kombu into one-inch squares with scissors. Soak the squares in a half water, half tamari soy sauce mixture (enough liquid to cover the kombu) for 1 to 2 days. Place them in an uncovered pot, add enough water/tamari soy sauce to cover, bring to a boil, immediately turn the flame to low, and place a heat deflector underneath. Slowly simmer for several hours, until most of the liquid has evaporated.

Shio kombu can be stored in a small jar. Since this condiment is very high in minerals, have only several pieces about twice a week.

## Nori Condiment

This condiment adds iron and other minerals to the diet and is milder than shio kombu.

*To prepare:*  Place 10 sheets of nori (broken into small pieces), 1 cup spring water, and 1/2 tablespoon of tamari soy sauce in a covered pot and bring to a boil. Turn the flame to low and slowly simmer for 20 to 30 minutes, or until most of the liquid has boiled away, leaving a paste of nori.

Store in a jar, and have several tablespoons two or three times per week with meals.

## Compresses, Body Scrubs, and Plasters ──────────

### Hot Water Body Scrub

A daily body scrub with a hot towel is a simple and effective way to promote overall health and vitality. It activates circulation, releases stagnation in the joints, and helps break down fats deposited under the skin.

After many years of consuming cheese, chicken, meat, eggs, and other animal foods, many people develop a layer of hard fat just below the skin. This condition occurs in thin people as well as in the overweight, and produces hard, dry skin and a reduced capacity to sweat.

The skin is one of the body's major organs of discharge. When the pores and sweat glands become constricted and blocked with fatty deposits, toxic factors that are normally discharged can start to accumulate. This can lead to the buildup of toxins throughout the body, creating a medium for the eventual development of arthritis and other degenerative conditions. It is therefore important to avoid the foods that cause these fats to develop and to practice daily body scrubbing in order to open the pores and allow excess to come out.

Body scrubbing can be done before or after a bath or shower.

*To do a body scrub:*  All you need is a sink with hot water and a medium-sized cotton towel. Turn the hot water on. Hold your towel

at either end and run the center part under the stream of hot water.
Wring the towel out, and, while it is still hot and steamy, begin to
scrub yourself with it.

Do a section of your body at a time, for example, beginning
with your hands and fingers, and working your way up the arms
to the shoulders, neck, and face, and then downward to the chest,
upper back, abdomen, lower back, buttocks, legs, feet, and toes.
Make sure to scrub your entire body so that the skin turns slightly
red or until each part becomes warm. You can reheat your towel
by running it under the hot water after doing each section or as
soon as it starts to cool.

A hot towel body scrub is ideal once or twice a day. When you do
it in the morning, it has the effect of vitalizing and energizing you for
the day's activity. When you do it in the evening, it releases stress
and tension and relaxes and refreshes you. The total body scrub only
takes about ten minutes to do.

## Hot Towel Compresses

Hot towels can also be used to relax specific areas of the body and
for the relief of aches, pains, and stiffness in the joints.

Prepare a hot towel as described above, fold it into sections, and
apply it hot to the area you wish to treat. Hold it in place until it
cools, and then reheat the towel and apply it again. Continue
applying the hot towel for five to ten minutes or until the area
becomes red or warm.

Hot towels, or other hot applications, should not be applied to
joints or other parts of the body that are hot, swollen, or inflamed.
Cool applications, such as tofu or green-vegetable plasters, are
better for easing discomfort produced by these conditions.

## Ginger Compress

Ginger compresses work like plain hot towels to stimulate circulation,
dissolve stagnation, and relax specific areas of the body. Adding
freshly grated ginger to the hot water makes the heat even more
stimulating and penetrating.

Ginger compresses can be done alone if you are able to reach the
area you wish to treat, or with a partner if the area is hard to reach.

*To make the compress:* You will need a medium-sized piece of
fresh ginger root (available at most natural food or Oriental mar-
kets), a flat metal grater, some cheesecloth, three medium-sized
cotton towels, and a medium- to large-sized pot with a lid.

Grate the ginger root on the metal grater and place a golf ball-sized clump in a double layer of cheesecloth. Tie the cheesecloth at the top to form a sack. Then, place a gallon of water in a pot and bring it up to but not over the boiling point. Just before the water starts to boil, turn the flame down to low.

Next, hold the sack over the pot and squeeze as much of the ginger juice as you can into the water. Then drop the sack in the pot. Make sure the water does not boil, as this will weaken the effect of the compress. Place the lid on the pot and let the ginger sack simmer in the water for about five minutes.

Then, fold one of the towels several times lengthwise, so that it becomes long and thin. Hold it from both ends and dip the center into the hot ginger water. Wring it out tightly, and if it is too hot to place on the skin, shake it slightly. Place the hot towel on the area you wish to treat, and place one of the dry towels on top of it to reduce heat loss.

While the hot towel is still on the skin, prepare another ginger towel in the manner described above. Apply it as soon as the first towel cools, and repeat this procedure, replacing towels every two to three minutes until the skin becomes red and warm.

The ginger compress is fine for use by normally healthy adults as a part of general health improvement. However, it should not be applied in cases of fever or inflammation. Persons with cancer or other serious illness should use a milder application, such as a hot-towel compress, unless otherwise advised by a qualified macrobiotic teacher. The ginger compress can be applied to loosen stagnation and dissolve hardening, as in hard, stiff, or tight joints. However, it should not be used on joints or other parts of the body that are hot, swollen, or inflamed.

### Ginger Body Scrub

A special body scrub can also be done with hot ginger water. Dip the towel in the pot of hot ginger water as described above, but instead of applying it to only one area, use it to scrub your entire body. It can be done after the ginger compress or by itself. Many people find plain hot water body scrubbing more convenient during the week, and use the ginger body scrub on the weekends when more time is available. One pot of hot ginger water can be used for two days of body scrubs. Simply reheat the water before using (do not bring it to a boil).

## Tofu Plaster

Raw tofu is milder, yet more effective than ice to draw out a fever or help ease swelling or inflammation in the joints.

*To prepare a tofu plaster:*   Squeeze the water from a block of tofu. Mash the tofu in a suribachi with about 10 to 20 percent whole wheat pastry flour and 5 percent freshly grated ginger. Mix thoroughly and place the tofu mixture about 1/2-inch thick on a clean piece of cotton cheesecloth or a cotton towel. Apply directly to the forehead, back of the head, or affected joint. Change every couple of hours or leave on until the tofu becomes warm or the temperature drops.

## Green Vegetable Plaster

Raw green vegetables can also be used to lower fevers or ease swelling and inflammation in the joints.

*To prepare:*   Chop a bunch of washed greens (such as collard, kale, or watercress) very finely. Place them in a suribachi and grind them thoroughly. If the greens are very watery, mix in a little pastry flour to hold the mixture together. Place the mashed greens on a piece of cotton cheesecloth or cotton linen to form a layer about 1/2-inch thick.

Apply directly to the forehead or other parts of the body. Change every several hours or leave on until the greens become warm.

## Tofu-Green Vegetable Plaster

This plaster combines the effects of raw tofu and greens and can also be used to bring down a fever or ease swelling and inflammation.

*To prepare:*   Chop a bunch of leafy greens very finely and mash in a suribachi. Place 1/2 pound of tofu and about 5 percent grated ginger in the suribachi and grind the ingredients into a thick paste. Place the paste on a clean piece of cotton cheesecloth or towel, creating a layer about 1/2-inch thick. Apply as above.

## Salt Pack

Roasted salt can be used to warm and soothe any part of the body, for example, the shoulders or lower back when aches and pains are felt there. It can also be applied to the abdomen to help relieve diarrhea or to ease menstrual cramps, but, as with other hot applications, should not be applied in cases of swelling, fever, or inflammation.

*To prepare:* Dry-roast salt in a stainless-steel skillet. Stir it from time to time until it becomes very hot. Place the hot salt in a *thick cotton* sack or pillowcase. Do not use a sack made of synthetic material, as the hot salt will cause it to melt. Tie the sack with a piece of string and then wrap it in a thick cotton bath towel.

Place it on the area you wish to treat, and leave it on until it cools. You may replace it with another salt pack if you wish, but one application is usually enough. Save the salt, as it can be re-roasted several more times. Discard it once it turns grey, as it will no longer hold heat at this point.

### Lotus Root Plaster

Freshly grated lotus root can be used to draw stagnated mucus from the sinuses, nose, throat, and bronchi.

*To prepare a plaster:* Wash a piece of lotus root and grate it on a flat metal grater. Mix the grated lotus with 10 to 15 percent whole wheat pastry flour and 5 percent freshly grated ginger. Spread a half-inch layer of this mixture onto a piece of cotton linen and apply so that the mixture comes into direct contact with the skin. Leave it on for several hours or overnight.

This plaster can be used daily for up to ten days, or until stagnated deposits of mucus begin to discharge. A hot ginger compress or hot water towels may be applied to the area before the lotus plaster is put on to warm the area and loosen stagnation.

### Dark Sesame Oil

Sesame oil can be used to keep the skin healthy and smooth. It is helpful in relieving minor burns or chapped skin.

*For burns:* First soak the area in cool salt water, then apply a piece of tofu until the pain is gone. Then, gently rub dark sesame oil on the area.

*For chapped skin:* Gently rub on the affected area when needed.

## Baths and Soaks

### Daikon Hip Bath

Reproductive disorders have become epidemic in modern society. According to present estimates, as many as one in five American couples is infertile. An estimated 40 percent of women have *Premenstrual Syndrome* (*PMS*), including 3 percent with severe cases. Forty percent of women have fibroid tumors. Annualy there are about 4.2 million operations on female genital organs, including about 700,000 hysterectomies. About 1 in 5 babies is delivered by Cesarean section.

The reproductive organs are a frequent site for the accumulation of excess. In women, these accumulations may take the form of fibroid tumors, dermoid cysts, or in extreme cases, cancer of the ovaries, uterus, or cervix. Vaginal discharge, a common condition today, is an indication that excess is beginning to accumulate throughout the body.

In traditional macrobiotic medicine, the daikon hip bath is frequently used to relieve female reproductive disorders. Ideally, the bath water should contain dried daikon leaves (turnip greens or arame sea vegetable can be used when daikon greens are not available).

*To prepare:*   Hang fresh leaves out of direct sunlight until they turn brown and brittle. Place about four to five bunches of dried leaves or a double handful of arame in a large pot. Add about four to five quarts of water and bring to a boil. Reduce the flame to medium and boil until the water turns brown. Add a handful of sea salt and stir well to dissolve.

Run hot water in the bathtub and add the mixture together with another large handful of sea salt. Add only enough water to cover the body from the waist down. Sit in the tub and cover your upper body with a thick cotton towel to prevent chills and absorb perspiration. If the water begins to cool, add more hot water and stay in the bath for ten to twelve minutes.

The hot bath will cause your lower body to become very red as a result of an increase in circulation. This, along with the heat will loosen fat and mucus deposits in the pelvic region.

Following the hip bath, douche with a special solution.

*To prepare:*   Squeeze the juice from half a lemon into warm bancha tea or add one to two teaspoons of brown rice vinegar to warm bancha tea. Add a three-finger pinch of sea salt, stir, and use as a douche. The douching solution helps dislodge deposits of mucus and fat that have been loosened during the bath.

The hip bath and douche can be repeated every day for up to ten days. During this time, it is important to eat well and to avoid foods that contribute to the buildup of excess in the reproductive tract and throughout the body, including in and around the joints.

### Daikon-Leaf Skin Wash

Dried daikon (or turnip) greens are also helpful in relieving skin conditions such as eczema, acne, impetigo, and others.

Prepare the dried leaves as indicated above. However, rather than pouring the mixture into the bathtub, dip a cotton towel into the pot and squeeze it lightly. Apply it to the affected area, making repeated applications until the skin turns red.

### Rice Bran (Nuka) Skin Wash or Bath

*Nuka,* or rice bran, can be purchased at most natural food stores. It has been used for centuries in traditional cultures to promote healthy skin and to improve skin disorders. Rice bran contains natural oil that helps the skin return to a smooth and healthy condition. The hair can also be washed in nuka water.

*To prepare a skin wash:* Wrap nuka in a cheesecloth sack. Place in warm water, squeeze, and shake. The nuka will dissolve and the water turn yellowish and a white foam may form on the surface. Lightly wash the affected area several times with a towel or face-cloth that has been dipped in the nuka water.

A person with skin problems can also take a bath in which nuka has been dissolved.

Put about 3 to 5 tablespoons of nuka into a white cotton sock or sack made of thin cotton cloth or cheesecloth. Tie the sack so that the nuka does not fall out. Place the sack in the bathwater and squeeze it until a milky liquid comes out. Mix the milky liquid in the water and use it to wash the skin, including the areas where the disorder is present.

If you cannot find rice bran, rolled oats can be substituted. About 1/4 cup can be used. Nuka or oat applications may also be used to ease the itching and discomfort of poison ivy or insect bites.

### Ginger Water Foot Soak

Often, years of consuming animal proteins and fats causes hard calluses to build up on the bottoms of the feet and toes. These deposits interfere with the smooth exchange of energy between the feet and the environment, especially the flow of energy that runs through the meridians that connect to the toes (see Chapter 7).

Soaking the feet in a pot of hot ginger water helps to soften these deposits and increases overall circulation. It can also help ease stiffness, pain, or tightness in the feet and toes. However, persons experiencing acute attacks of gout or swelling and inflammation in the feet are advised to wait until a more normal condition is reestablished before using the ginger foot soak.

It can be done immediately after a ginger compress or bodyscrub by placing both feet in the pot of hot ginger water. Let the feet soak for five to ten minutes, then rub briskly with a dry cotton towel.

# 7. Arthritis and Body Energy

Many thousands of years ago, ancient healers perceived the unity
between man, nature, and energy. They developed a vast cosmology
that explained the creation of the universe, out of which the understanding of health and sickness evolved.

Underlying their view was the understanding that all things were
manifestations of energy. In ancient China, this energy was given the
name *Ch'i*. In Japan it was named *Ki*, and in India, *prana*. All things
in nature—from the largest galaxy to the tiniest atom—were seen as
manifestations of this universal energy.

An awareness of the human body as energy underlies the practice
of acupuncture, herbal medicine, palm healing, massage, and other
traditional healing arts. In the twentieth century, modern physics
arrived at essentially the same conclusion regarding the nature of the
material world: that matter is nothing but moving, vibrating energy.

In Japan, even today, the word Ki is used often in everyday
language. Sickness, for example, is referred to as *Byo Ki*, or "suffering ki." *Ku Ki*, or the "ki of emptiness," means "air," while *Yu Ki*,
or "active ki," means "courage," Hundreds of other examples exist,
showing how deeply ingrained this concept has become in the Oriental
way of thinking.

The understanding of man is also influenced by this concept. In
Japanese, for example, the word for human being is *Hito*. The word
is a combination of the syllables *Hi*, which means "sun" or "fire," and
*To*, which means "spirit." This word implies that the human body,
mind, and spirit are one, and are manifestations of highly charged,
radiant energy.

The energy that animates all of our life functions originates outside the body in the surrounding environment. Our body constantly
receives energy from stars, galaxies, constellations, planets, and from
the universe itself. These, and other forms of energy that originate
in the cosmos, are referred to in macrobiotics as "heaven's force."
Meanwhile, the earth—a huge spinning mass that moves through
space with enormous speed—generates energy of its own. These
powerful centrifugal forces arise largely as the result of the earth's
rotation, and are referred to as "earth's force."

Incoming forces from the universe enter the body through the top
of the head, in the region of the hair spiral, or cowlick. (This spiral
is a reflection of the pattern of movement of this cosmic force.) After

entering the head, heaven's force proceeds downward through the body, and exits in the region of the sexual organs. Meanwhile, earth's force enters the body in the region of the sexual organs and moves upward, exiting the body through the hair spiral. These upward and downward currents run along a central line of energy. This central channel carries the primary charge that creates "aliveness," animating all of the body's functions and supplying every cell with the energy needed for life.

At certain places along this central line, heaven's and earth's forces intersect and create highly charged spirals. Five of these "colliding places" of energy arise within the body, and when counted along with the two regions where these forces enter and leave the body, produce what ancient Aryuvedic doctors referred to as the seven *chakras* or "wheels" of energy.

The chakras supply energy to the organs, glands, cells, and tissues. The seventh chakra at the top of the head, for example, charges the right and left hemispheres of the brain, as does the sixth, or midbrain chakra located deep within the brain. The fifth, or throat chakra, energizes the thyroid and parathyroid glands, as well as the vocal cords, while the heart and lungs are activated primarily by the fourth, or heart chakra, deep in the center of the chest. The organs in the central part of the body—the stomach, spleen, pancreas, liver, and gall bladder—are especially charged by the third, or stomach chakra in the solar plexus. The second, or hara chakra, located deep within the small intestine, activates the small and large intestine and kidneys, while the first, or sexual chakra, charges the bladder and reproductive organs.

If we compare the central line to a mighty river, then the chakras are like powerful whirlpools that arise within the ongoing stream of energy. Meanwhile, the flowing river branches off into smaller streams, known as *meridians*, that run just below the skin. The meridians branch out from the central channel in the way that the ridges of a pumpkin branch from its central core.

Each meridian continuously subdivides into smaller and smaller branches, which ultimately connect with the smallest biological units of the body: the cells. In other words, each cell is constantly supplied with energy by the meridians, which in turn receive energy from the central channel and chakras. Energy also flows in the opposite direction: from the cells to the meridians, and then to the central channel and chakras. The human body is composed of an intricate network of energy currents that charge all of its functions.

Health depends on the body's ability to conduct this life energy. If the flow of energy through the cells, tissues, and organs becomes overactive on the one hand, or underactive and stagnant on the other, imbalance or sickness is the result.

How the body conducts life energy depends on the quality of the other major stream that nourishes it: that of the blood and body fluids. The quality of blood and body fluids is determined largely by what we eat and drink. If the quality of food is well balanced, then the flow of energy through the cells, organs, meridians, and chakras occurs smoothly.

Extreme foods create imbalance in the body's energy flow. Meat, eggs, poultry, cheese, and other animal products create a fatty condition in the bloodstream. Fats interfere with the smooth exchange of nutrients and energy between the blood and cells. Cells also become encased in a layer of fat and mucus as the result of overconsuming these foods, and this diminishes their conductivity. It can also block the smooth release of energy and waste products, causing excess to accumulate and energy to stagnate.

On the other hand, simple sugars, such as those in refined sugar, honey, maple syrup, chocolate, carob, and tropical fruits, enter the bloodstream too rapidly. This causes a quick rise in the level of blood sugar and a rapid burst of metabolic activity in the cells. This active energy is short lived, however, and can exhaust and deplete the vitality of the cells, while producing an accumulation of toxic waste.

A diet that is high in calories causes the body's metabolic activity to become continuously overactive. Excessive energy is constantly produced in the cells and discharged through the meridians and chakras. This can interfere with the flow of energy in the other direction—from the primary channel and chakras to the meridians, organs, and cells, resulting in diminished sensitivity to environmental energies. Moreover, the continuous production of waste from an extreme diet overloads the body's discharge systems, leading eventually to the accumulation of toxins throughout the body, including in the bones and joints.

During the embryonic period when the body is forming, energy from the environment charges its innermost regions. Here it creates compact energy spirals that eventually develop into organs, and then flows out through the front of the body. The energy that forms the lungs, heart, large and small intestine is discharged upward, forming parallel streams that later become the arms. The energy that creates the liver, gall bladder, kidneys, bladder, stomach, spleen, and pancreas is discharged downward, forming parallel streams that become the legs.

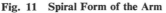

**Fig. 11   Spiral Form of the Arm**

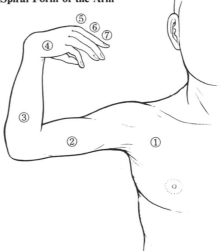

Each logarithmic orbit of
the spiral developed later as
a section of the arm. The
tip of the fingers are the
most inner part of the spiral.

These parallel streams curl inward, forming contracted spirals.
Joints are the regions that divide one orbit from the next in these
spiral formations. The first orbit of the arm spiral—the root of the
arm—includes the shoulder blade and arm socket. The second orbit
is comprised of the area that extends from the shoulder to the elbow;
the thrid, the area from the elbow to the wrist; the fourth, the region
from the wrist to the knuckles; the fifth, the first section of the
fingers; the sixth, the second, or middle section of the fingers; and
the seventh, the third and last section of the fingers.

A similar pattern develops in the legs, feet, and toes. This spiral
pattern contains seven complete stages, or orbits, reflecting the pattern of creation found throughout the universe. Spiral forms exist
everywhere—from huge galactic whirlpools to the movements of
preatomic particles. Nature is comprised of a multitude of spirals
large and small.

In our bodies, for example, hair spirals around a central point, the
crown. The ear is also formed in spirallic orbits, while the eyes are
a series of concentric orbits that include the white of the eye, the
iris, and the pupil, which expands and contracts in a spiral motion.
The human breast is a spiral ending in a central point, the nipple;
while the layers of the brain are arranged in a spiral around the
central midbrain. Other spirals are not visible to the naked eye but
can be seen with microscopes. These include the intertwining coils of
DNA found in the nucleus of the cell.

Science is beginning to recognize this universal pattern, as the following quote, taken from the March 30, 1988, issue of the *Berkshire Eagle*, illustrates.

> *Scientists tackle spiral riddle.*   Los Angeles (UPI)—DNA, the master molecule of life, is a spiraling ladder loaded with the hereditary characters that determine everything from the color of eyes to the shape of a leaf. On a larger scale, spirals are the shapes of whirlpools and tornadoes, and on Jupiter, a spiral is the form of the whirling Great Red Spot.
>
> Scientists, mindful that galaxies, the most titanic spirals of all, did not take shape by accident, now think they were formed by electromagnetic forces that whipped cosmic matter into one of the most widely repeated forms in nature. "Vortices," theoretical physicist Anthony Peratt said of spiral shapes, "are important in nature from the smallest imaginable to the largest. Water draining from a bathtub forms a vortex. Vortices are morphologies (structures) that can be seen everywhere."

As we saw above, the arms and legs were formed out of energy spirals. Now let us see how individual meridians are also formed in spirals, and how this pattern of development is related to the function of the joints. We can consider the heart meridian as a typical example.

The heart meridian begins in the region of the heart chakra. In actuality, it is connected to a spinal vertabrae behind the chakra. It is here that the environmental energy linked to the heart meridian enters the body during the embryonic period. Thus the starting point of the meridian is actually a joint. From here, the meridian divides into the following sections:

1.  From the heart chakra it continues to the shoulder. At the shoulder there is a joint.
2.  From the shoulder, it runs down the arm to the elbow, where another joint develops.
3.  From the elbow, the meridian continues down the forearm to the wrist, forming another section. The wrist is a joint.
4.  From the wrist it continues to the knuckle, or base of the little finger, forming another section. Here there is another joint.
5.  From the base of the little finger, it continues up to the first joint, forming another section. Again we have another division ending in a joint.
6.  The meridian continues to the second joint of the little finger. Another section, another joint.

7.  The meridian then continues to the fingertip.

The heart meridian can be divided into seven sections, as can the arm as a whole. This spiral starts with the largest loop—which originates in the center of the body—and continues to shorten as it moves toward the periphery, ending in the shortest section, the fingertip. The meridian spiral begins with a joint—the spinal vertabrae—and at each change to a smaller loop there is also a joint. When the meridian spiral changes from one loop to the next, points of highly charged energy develop, eventually forming joints. Other meridians—including those that flow downward into the legs and feet—also have the same general pattern.

Are there other structures in nature that have a similar form? Since the order of the universe exists in all things, we should be able to find similar patterns everywhere. Plants, for example, have the same general pattern of development, as the structure of a tree reveals. Each of the junctions where a tree branches out toward the periphery is equivalent to a joint in the human body. However, the divisions of the tree are solid and fixed, while in human beings the joints are flexible and mobile. Moreover, the roots of the tree are deep within the ground, and the tree receives strong energy from the earth, while the root of the human joint system—the spine—receives strong energy from heaven. These differences reflect the complementarity that exists between plants and animals.

## Energy Patterns in Arthritis

Specifically then, how can we use this understanding to help solve the problem of arthritis? The basic aspect of arthritis, problems in the joints, can occur in widely dispersed areas of the body. Arthritis is an indication that the flow of energy through the meridians has become unbalanced, and that other parts of the body, especially the internal organs, are also affected. As we saw above, the joints are areas that divide the spiral orbits of the arms and legs. They are concentrated gathering places of energy. Normally, each joint is capable of a wide range of movement. Their movements can be divided into basic stages that correspond to the cycle of energy described in Chapter 3:

1.  *Upward motion:* such as when a joint is stretched upward or outward.
2.  *Expanding motion:* such as the active expansion and contraction that occurs in the joints during vigorous movement.

3. *Downward motion:* such as when the joints return to a more stable or balanced position after vigorous exertion.
4. *Condensed motion:* including when they become fixed or contracted as a result of bearing weight or pushing a heavy object.
5. *Floating motion:* including more relaxed, flexible movements.

All of the joints in the body have these five abilities. Joints at the periphery of the body, such as the fingers, have greater flexibility and capacity for refined movement, while those in the lower or central part of the body are able to bear more weight and are responsible for larger body movements.

In arthritis, the joints lose their natural flexibility and range of motion. Hardness, stiffness, or tightness indicates that blockage or stagnation has developed in the flow of energy along the meridians. The primary cause of this condition is the overintake of foods with strong contracting energy, including meat, poultry, hard cheese, eggs, salt, and hard baked flour products. As the tendons and ligaments that connect the bones become tighter and more constricted, energy can no longer flow smoothly through the joint.

Swelling and inflammation indicate that energy in the meridians has become overactive, and is gathering in the joints. The overintake of sugar, tropical fruits and vegetables, chocolate, and other foods with expanding energy, as well as too much fat and liquid, can produce this condition. As the tendons and ligaments expand and become

**Fig. 12A   The Correspondence between the Meridians and the Fingers and Toes**

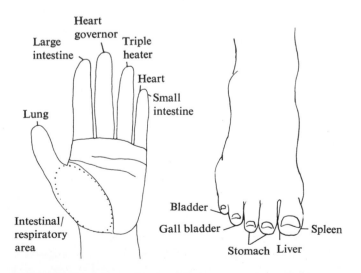

**Fig. 12B  Beginning of the Kidney
Meridian (Yu-Sen)**

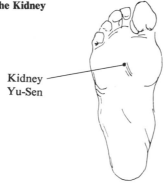

Kidney
Yu-Sen

swollen, the joint becomes painful, its range of motion diminishes, and it is less able to bear weight.

The location of the disorder indicates which part of the body's energy system is most affected. Each of the fingers and toes, for example, corresponds to a specific meridian and organ. The wrists, elbows, shoulders, knees, and ankles also have meridan and organ correspondences. Correspondences between the fingers, toes, and meridians and organs are presented in the diagram above. However, please note that the middle and ring fingers are connected to meridians that arise directly from the chakras—especially the heart, stomach, and small intestine (hara) chakras—rather than from specific organs.

These meridians are referred to in Oriental medicine as the heart governor and triple heater. They regulate comprehensive bodily functions such as the circulation of blood and body fluids (in the case of the heart governor) and the generation of heat and metabolic energy (in the case of the triple heater).

Let us now consider how these correspondences work in the case of arthritis. As we can see in the diagram, the index finger is part of the large intestine meridian. Swelling in the joints of the index finger indicates that energy in the large intestine meridian has become overactive. This condition corresponds to imbalance in the large intestine itself, so that overactivity and swelling in the peripheral meridian and joint usually mean some degree of swelling or overactivity is taking place in the organ. These imbalances may produce symptoms such as digestive upsets, diahrrea, or, if the swelling of the intestinal lining becomes chronic, constipation.

These conditions are usually not associated with problems in the joints, but as we can see, they are intimately connected. The body is an interconnected whole. Let us now see how the types of arthritis introduced in the previous chapters correspond to disorders deep within the body.

*Rheumatoid Arthritis.* The primary symptoms of rheumatoid arthritis—swelling, pain, and inflammation in the knuckles, wrists, knees, and ball of the foot—indicate an overactive condition in the meridians. When swelling or inflammation occurs in the joints of the fingers, the following organs and functions are affected:

| Finger | Meridain/Organ/Chakra |
| --- | --- |
| Base of thumb | Lung and its functions |
| Index | Large intestine and its functions |
| Middle | Heart, stomach, and small intestine (hara) chakras; especially their function in regulating the circulation of blood and body fluids |
| Ring | Heart, stomach, and small intestine (hara) chakras; especially their function in generating heat and metabolic energy |
| Fifth finger (pinky) | Heart, small intestine, and their functions |

If the wrist is the primary joint affected with rheumatoid arthritis, the functions of the heart, small intestine, lungs, large intestine, and three chakras are affected. When this form of arthritis strikes the knees, the functions of the liver, spleen, gall bladder, stomach, bladder, and kidneys are also compromised. If the inside of the knee is most affected, the related organ dysfunction is located primarily in the spleen, liver, kidneys, and pancreas, while if the outside or front portion of the knee is most affected, organ dysfunction is more pronounced in the stomach and gall bladder. Pain or swelling in the ball of the foot corresponds to dysfunction in the kidney, spleen, and liver.

*Lupus and Arthritis.* Lupus, with its wide range of symptoms, indicates disorder throughout the network of meridians, organs, and chakras. Pain in the knuckles can indicate dysfunction in any of the organs or chakra functions listed above, and frequently correlates with the symptoms that accompany lupus. Inflammation in the pleural lining, for example, indicates overactivity in the lung meridian, while inflammation in the area around the heart indicates that the heart,

heart governor, and triple heater meridians are dysfunctioning. These internal conditions often appear as arthritis in the corresponding fingers.

Arthritis in the index and fifth fingers indicates overactivity in the large and small intestine, which correlates with possible swelling in the lining of the abdominal cavity and digestive disturbances. Overactivity in the heart governor and triple heater meridians, reflected in the middle and ring finger, can produce discoloration in the face, especially in the cheeks and across the bridge of the nose.

When arthritis develops in the inside or back portion of the knee, the functions of the kidneys, bladder, liver, spleen, and pancreas are affected; while arthritis in the outer or front portion of the knee indicates a greater degree of dysfunction in the stomach and gall bladder. Symptoms such as mouth ulcers and loss of protein in the urine, which often accompany lupus, are reflections of the involvement these organs.

*Osteoarthritis.* The formation of bony nodes in the fingers that occurs in osteoarthritis indicates that the flow of energy through the meridians has become stagnant. Accumulation of protein, fats, and minerals in the joints—resulting from overintake of animal food—reflects a parallel buildup in the internal organs, as well as in the arteries and blood vessels. The location of these deposits can be determined by seeing which fingers are affected. (Please refer to the chart above.) For example, nodes in the fifth finger indicate the buildup of fat and cholesterol in the heart and small intestine, while nodes appearing on the middle finger indicate that deposits are also forming throughout the circulatory system.

Osteoarthritis of the spine is an indication that the flow of energy through the primary channel and chakras has become stagnant. If hardening occurs in the upper spine, the functioning of the heart and lungs has been affected. Hardening in the middle spine indicates greater involvement of the stomach, spleen, pancreas, liver, gall bladder, and kidneys; while hardening in the lower spine is an indication of trouble in the small and large intestines, bladder, and reproductive organs.

Osteoarthritis in the knee or hip is an indication of stagnation in the liver and gall bladder meridians, and may indicate the accumulation of fat in these organs, with the possible formation of gallstones. The spleen, pancreas, kidney, and bladder may also be accumulating fats, with the possible development of stones, cysts, or tumors in these organs.

108

*Ankylosing Spondylitis.* The hardening of the spine in ankylosing spondylitis is an indication that energy is not flowing smoothly through the primary channel and chakras. Hardening in the lower spine correlates with blockages of energy (often taking the form of fat and cholesterol deposits) in the bladder, sexual organs—including the prostate gland and uterus—and the small and large intestine.

As hardening progresses upward along the spine, energy in the corresponding chakras and organs becomes increasingly stagnant. If the condition reaches the stage where the spine remains permanently bent, the flow of heaven's and earth's forces through the primary channel may diminish to the point of not actively charging the body's activities and functions.

*Gout.* The predominant area where gout strikes—the base of the large toe—is a region where three meridians meet. The kidney meridian begins near the base of the large toe on the bottom of the foot (see above diagram), and runs from here up along the inside of the leg. The symptoms of gout indicate trouble in the kidney meridian and kidneys. The excessive intake of animal protein, a primary contributor to gout, creates acidic byproducts that overwork and stress the kidneys while overconsumption of animal fat often leads to the formation of fatty deposits, further diminishing kidney function.

Moreover, continual consumption of icy cold drinks—also a factor in gout—can cause these deposits to calcify and condense into stones. Accumulation of fat and mucus in the kidneys is also accelerated by overintake of sugar, honey, concentrated sweeteners, tropical fruits, and ice cream, and by intake of rich, creamy sauces, desserts, and oily or greasy foods.

The meridians of the liver and spleen also meet in the region of the large toe. The dietary excesses that contribute to gout also affect these organs. Overconsumption of alcohol, for example, weakens the liver and contributes to gout, while fatty animal foods—including dairy products—often cause stagnation in the spleen and lymphatic system, a condition that underlies many cases of gout.

## Balancing Meridian Energy

A balanced natural diet is the most fundamental way of avoiding the excesses that lead to imbalance in the organs, meridians, and joints. Arthritis is a preventable disease. Moreover, returning to a balanced diet—in combination with proper activity and way of life—can lead to restoration of a normal condition in the joints and meridians, even after the imbalance of arthritis has developed.

As we saw in Chapter 2, arthritis is considered an incurable disease. Modern treatments aim at controlling or minimizing symptoms, but the overall course of the disease remains unchanged. In order to fundamentally change an arthritic condition to a condition of normal, healthy balance, the factors that cause the disease—daily diet and way of life—need to be changed. Re-establishing balance in these aspects of life is the essence of the macrobiotic approach.

Along with this basic approach, supplementary methods can help establish balance in the flow of energy through the meridians and joints, and restore the body to a more normal degree of flexibility. In the following section, we introduce a simple series of exercises for stretching and energizing the meridians. These exercises are adapted from the traditional practice of *Do-In*, or natural self-massage and movement. Additional exercises are presented in my book, the *Book of Do-In: Exercise for Physical and Spiritual Development*, Japan Publications, 1979.

Persons with arthritis or other crippling diseases are of course advised to adapt any exercise program to their individual condition and abilities. It is further recommended that persons with more serious conditions contact their physician or other health professional when considering the advisability of beginning this or any other program of exercise or movement.

## Meridian Exercises

### 1. For the lung and large intestine

Begin by standing with feet slightly apart, about shoulder width. Bring the hands behind the back and lock the thumbs together. The fingers can be curled into a fist. From this beginning position, raise the arms back away from the body and at the same time look upward toward the ceiling, arching the spine backwards. This motion pushes the chest forward and stretches the middle organs and abdomen.

From this posture, bend in the opposite direction—forward from the hips—and stretch as far forward as comfortably possible. Let the arms follow this entire motion with hands remaining clasped, so that a full stretch of the arms is experienced. When done properly, the legs and spine form a 90-degree angle. Hold this forward bent position for two long, slow breaths, then return to an upright position. Release the thumbs and allow the hands to hang freely from the sides. This stretch may then be repeated.

This stretch activates the energy flow and physical function of the lungs and large intestine.

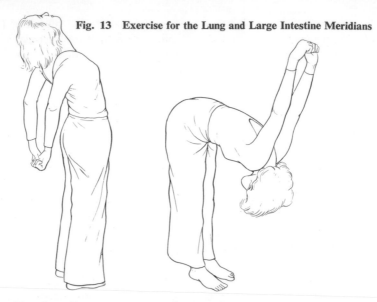

Fig. 13    Exercise for the Lung and Large Intestine Meridians

## 2.  For the spleen, pancreas, and stomach

Begin by sitting in what is called *seiza*, that is, with the legs folded under so the buttocks are sitting on the heels. This position, for some, may be an exercise in itself because of stiffness in the ankle and knee joints. In the seiza posture, clasp the hands together, intertwining the fingers. Then, slowly and smoothly, extend the arms and raise them until they are vertically aligned to the body.

Continue this stretching motion so that the body begins to stretch backward. This backward motion should continue until the torso stretches so that the head and shoulders, and then the spine, rest on the ground. Try to keep the legs firmly folded in the seiza position. If possible, the knees should remain touching the floor. Hold this position for two long, slow breaths. Then, reverse the motion and return to an erect posture, bringing the hands back to the lap. This stretch can be repeated again.

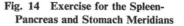
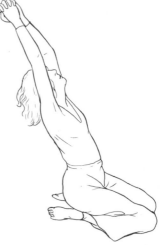

Fig. 14    Exercise for the Spleen-Pancreas and Stomach Meridians

This stretch activates the energy flow and physical functions of the stomach, spleen, and pancreas.

### 3. For the heart and small intestine

Begin by sitting on the floor. The feet are brought together so that the soles of the feet are touching each other. Both hands can firmly clasp the feet. This position extends the legs out at an angle with the knees bent. The knees should be touching the floor. Slowly, bring the feet, bottoms remaining clasped together, in toward the body. This strongly stretches the inner area of the thigh.

When the heels of the feet have been brought in as closely as comfortably possible, bend the torso forward, with the goal of bringing the forehead in contact with the hands. This forward bending motion should be accomplished from the hips to fully stretch the whole torso. Once the forehead touches the hands, maintain this posture for two long, slow breaths, then reverse the motion and straighten the body so that it returns to a vertical, sitting posture. Repeat the stretch again.

This stretch activates the energy flow and physical functions of the heart and small intestine.

**Fig. 15   Exercise for the Heart and Small Intestine Meridians**

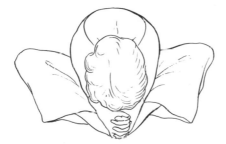

### 4. For the kidneys and bladder

Begin by sitting on the floor with legs together and fully extended forward so that the backs of the legs are touching the floor from the heel to the buttocks. Grasp the toes with each hand, slowly bending the body forward from the hips so as to stretch the entire spine. If possible, bring the forehead in contact with the knees.

Hold this position for two long, slow breaths, then raise the torso away from the legs, straightening the spine and returning to an erect sitting posture. The hands can relax and release their grip on the toes. Repeat the stretch.

This exercise activates the energy flow and physical functions of the kidneys and bladder.

112

Fig. 16   Exercise for the Kidney and Bladder Meridians

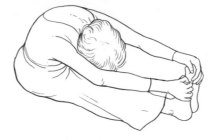

### 5.   For the heart governor and triple heater

Begin by sitting in the lotus position on the floor. The legs are crossed so the ankles can rest on the upper part of the thighs, one ankle on top of the other. From this lotus position, extend each arm and grasp the *opposite* knee with the hand. The right hand will be on top of the left knee and the left hand will be on top of the right knee. Bend forward slowly until the forehead touches the ground. Hold this position for two long, slow breaths. Then reverse the motion and raise the torso, returning it to an erect, sitting position. The lotus position can be changed, alternating one leg on top of the other, and the stretch can be repeated.

This exercise activates the energy flow and related functions of the triple heater and heart governor.

Fig. 17   Exercise for the Heart Governor and Triple Heater Meridians

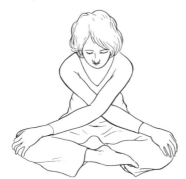
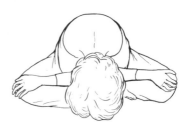

### 6.   For the liver and gall bladder

Begin by sitting on the floor. Extend  your legs forward with the backs of the legs firmly on the floor from the heels to the buttocks. The toes point up. Move the legs apart as far as possible while keeping them attached to the floor. With both hands, reach forward

and grasp one foot. Extend the spine from the hips so that the forehead touches the knee. Hold the position for two long, slow breaths.
Then return to an upright, erect posture.

Repeat this same motion with the opposite leg, grasping the toes
with both hands and stretching the torso forward so that the forehead touches the knees. Hold for two long, slow breaths, then slowly
return to an upright posture. Repeat the stretch to both sides.
This exercise activates the energy flow and physical functions of the
liver and gall bladder.

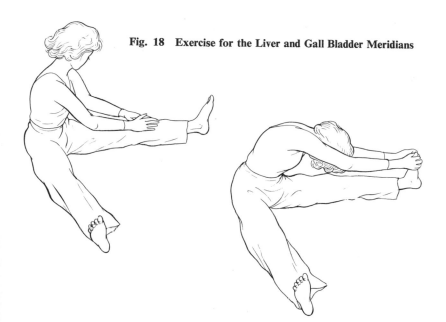

**Fig. 18   Exercise for the Liver and Gall Bladder Meridians**

# 8. Personal Experiences ▬▬

## Laureen Masini, Arlington, Virginia ▬▬▬▬▬

As a New York fashion model and eventually director of one of the largest modeling and self-improvement schools in the world, I had always been interested in food and health and nutrition. I had never eaten meat of any kind, and felt I was getting an excellent and balanced diet—since I ate seafood, whole grain bread, lots of fresh fruit and vegetables and salads.

About fifteen years ago I entered the travel business and began to travel worldwide, which made it difficult to follow a properly balanced food plan. White sugar, which I had always avoided, began to creep into my daily meals, as it was very difficult to resist the scrumptious pastries and desserts offered at almost every meal.

My first concern was the realization that I had started to put on weight and began to notice, mostly in the mornings, pains in my elbows and hips. I attributed it to fatigue due to the hectic pace of my work, but as the symptoms got worse I became alarmed, because by this time when I awoke in the mornings I felt that someone had my hips in a vise, and each day it seemed to be getting tighter and tighter.

I consulted a doctor who told me that I had arthritis and that it was not an unusual condition as people grew older. He suggested a prescription to relieve the pains. I felt that this was not a logical solution to my problem. What he offered was treatment of the symptoms but not any advice for the cause of the problem.

I was afraid and really alarmed as by now my right shoulder was also involved and I could not longer zip up the back of my skirt. I increased my intake of dairy products to at least two quarts of milk a day and lots of cheese. Things just got worse. I packed a little suitcase and said to my husband, "When the pain gets really bad, just take me to the hospital and forget me!"

That very afternoon, it was a Sunday in June, 1983, I decided I needed some more cheese so we drove to the health food store. The cheese man was busy so I browsed around the book department, and my eyes fell on Dr. Sattilaro's book, *Recalled by Life*. It was the story of a medical doctor who was dying of cancer and who, in the terminal stages, turned to macrobiotics.

The story fascinated me and gave me hope that each and every one

of us can make changes and take control of our health and our life.
I purchased all the books on macrobiotics that I could find; stories of
recoveries of terminally ill people who had turned to the macrobiotic way of life, and all the books written by Michio Kushi and his
wife Aveline.

I started to cook (which I had never liked) since there were no
cooking classes available at that time of the year. I also went for a
private educational interview with a macrobiotic teacher. This is
*very important*, as each person needs a food program that is planned
according to his or her individual problems. Within a few weeks
I began to notice a dramatic change in my physical condition. The
pains gradually began to disappear. My weight started to return to
normal and today I weight exactly what I weighed when I modeled.

I have taken responsibility and control over my health, and this
feeling of being in charge and not depending upon others cannot be
described except by saying it is the most thrilling experience of my
life. Because I now know that the philosophy of macrobiotic living is
the solution to the problems that every one of us faces. It puts each
of us in charge of our own life, and adds wonderful years to what is
often called the best years of our life.

## Janet Erickson, Minnetonka, Minnesota ———————

My medical diagnosis included degenerative arthritis of the hands,
hips, and knees. I was told by my doctor to go home and take aspirin
to treat the pain, and that there was no cure for my condition. "When
it becomes bad enough," he said, "we will do a knee and/or hip
replacement." I though this was the only option open to me until
I was introduced to macrobiotics, even though, deep down inside,
perhaps due to college exposure to some nutrition courses, I suspected
food helped or hindered my pain, physically and mentally.

I was aware that salt and packaged foods caused bloating and thus
more pain. Also, I noted my mood swings seemed to tie in with my
diet. Sugar and simple carbohydrates resulted in immediate "up"
moods, only to swing far "down" after they were over. What's more,
my father's and paternal grandmother's deaths from lung cancer
puzzled me. Neither smoked or drank liquor. Both lived in the
northern part of Maine. Why, then, did they die of lung cancer?
After reading the book, *Recalled by Life*, by Dr. Anthony Sattilaro,
and learning something about macrobiotics, the cancer deaths of my
father and grandmother, and my own arthritis seemed most logical to
me. I became willing to try and help myself. However first let me give
you a little of my own background.

however. Fifty-three years ago, I began having severe leg aches, called "growing pains" or rheumatism at that time. My parents and the doctors said "No" to my taking acrobatic and ballet lessons. Resentment entered my life at a very early age.

I was not a good eater, about the only thing I would eat was oatmeal, bananas, and white toast for the first five years of my life. From age five to twenty-one, eggs and fish—both shellfish and other types—became regular foods in my diet. I ate very little fruit and almost no vegetables. But daily I devoured cake, cookies, and pies. At age twenty-one, I married and moved from the East coast to the Midwest. Beef, and plenty of it, replaced fish. Eggs and chicken were eaten in great quantities. Weight gain followed.

With a "calorie conscious" background, I cut out the beef, and practically lived on chicken and eggs, bread and rolls. I eliminated the desserts but added alcohol in increasing amounts. Physically, I was active, cleaning first a six-room house and later a thirteen-room house, plus running after three children. I took some ballet lessons at age thirty-six when I enrolled my daughters. At age thirty-eight I took up tennis. And yes, I ached and hurt, physically and mentally. Aspirin and valium became a regular part of my daily diet.

At age forty-two, with the aid of three-hundred-and-fifty valium, I tried to commit suicide. I had lost all independence and had no mental control. Depression had turned to despair. Antidepressants were introduced. I lost my tonsils at age ten, my appendix at age twenty-three (two years after all my beef eating), and at age thirty-three my ovaries. Endometriosis, I was told. At age forty I had a tendon operation on my right knee.

For four years, from age forty-two until age forty-six, I was taking major tranquilizers and alcohol in increasing amounts, as well as popping valium. There were three more trips to the phsychiatric ward before I was treated for alcoholism in 1974 at the age of forty-six. Since then, I have not had any alcohol, but for two years after treatment I ate candy bars whenever I wanted to drink—which was often each and every day. I continued chicken, egg, potato, and bread eating, with few vegetables and fewer fruits, and almost no citrus—it always upset my stomach.

At age forty-two I had to quit tennis. My hands were too affected by arthritis and my knees were swelling and in pain. Until two plus years ago, my only physical activity from forty-two years of age was a six-month stint of swimming—ear infection took me out of the water—and a year of regular walking at a sports and health club. Using the nautilus equipment caused too much pain. When I started

to take ballroom dancing lessons, in the fall of 1984, I lived in fear of
having to give it up. My knees and hips, particularly, hurt, and of
course the knees were swelling badly.

In October of 1985 I met with Michio Kushi. I was told to look
at my hands—chicken hands—that is what I saw! I was to eat no
more chicken and no more eggs! The first eight weeks I was on a
specially adjusted variation of the standard macrobiotic diet. After
four weeks, the pain and swelling in my hands and knees was much
better. Going up and down stairs was no longer painful. After eight
weeks I lost excess weight. I had energy galore. I felt mentally alert,
very positive, and very "upbeat." There were no more wide mood
swings. My digestive system felt the best I can remember. I had no
more bouts with constipation. I was taking no medication.

I took three series of cooking classes and enjoyed macrobiotic
dinner parties. I felt good in every way. A little thing, like dealing
cards for bridge, changed from being very painful to pain free. Much
gratitude. I had a total sense of well-being, physically, mentally, and
spiritually. And I am now dancing up a storm!

Why, then, did I experiment with the macrobiotic diet? Primarily to
test any correlation between foods eaten and arthritis pain. In other
words, does the macrobiotic diet really make a difference or was it
all in my head? A hot fudge sundae with salted peanuts left me with
an upset stomach, as well as pain in my hands, swelling and pain in
my left knee. Mentally and energywise I was a mess. I was quickly
convinced that food caused my arthritis and could also control it.

I have continued to experiment, less drastically, to find my level of
variance while maintaining physical and mental comfort. Whenever
I go too far, I return to a simple diet and within twenty-four hours
I feel balanced again. It takes longer for the arthritic pain to completely go away. No one knows better than I how I feel.

A doctor (who knew I was eating macrobiotically and was worried
about my weight loss) insisted I have a blood test immediately to
check for anemia, potassium and calcium levels and whatever else
I don't know. Two days later the doctor called to give me a 100
percent grade of health. It cost me money to hear what I already
knew!

**Beverly Lemar (by Cynthia Smith)** ───────────────────

At just over five-feet tall, Beverly Lemar's dark, honey-colored hair
and cute, pixie-like face light up a room. There is an air of excited
energy about her, as if her personality voltage is tuned up an extra

notch. Looking years younger than her age of forty-one, there is little to show that Beverly, less than a year-and-a-half ago, nearly died of a disease she had never heard of before. This is the story of her struggle and victory over that disease.

For most of her life, Beverly experienced sickness as something that happened to other people. She rarely got colds, flu, headaches or other maladies that plague most of us. That changed however in 1983, when at thirty-six, she began experiencing some strange sensations in her body. Her hands began to swell and her fingers stiffened; she was feeling unusually tired and was cold most of the time. She took some time off from her job as auditor with human services for the state of Maine, but the symptoms persisted. Exhausted and unable to get a full night's sleep, Beverly began searching for the answer to her debilitating condition.

After visiting numerous doctors and receiving diverse opinions about her condition, Beverly was finally diagnosed as having *Scleroderma*, a form of arthritis. Translated literally, Scleroderma means "hard skin," and little is known why it causes an overproduction of *collagen*, the body's connective tissue, and results in a thickening and hardening of the skin. In its advanced stages, the internal organs and body become rigid and atrophy. Over 500,000 Americans, mostly middle-aged women, suffer from this disease. Over half of the patients with advanced Scleroderma die within seven years.

As Beverly's condition rapidly weakened over the next seven months, she was forced to take a leave of absence from her job, and at one point was hospitalized. A numbness eventually spread over her arms and legs, and she became unable to feed and clothe herself. Her weight dropped to 85 pounds. Her skin had toughened like an alligator hide, and her armpits and neck had fused to the rest of her body. "It was the most horrible thing you could imagine," Beverly explained. "My body just slowly hardened and thickened before my eyes and I lost all the feeling in it." Eventually she had trouble breathing, and digesting her food, and was told by her doctor not to be too optimistic about the future.

Beverly had been to a nutritionist in the early stages of her illness who recommended a complete change in her diet, lifestyle and thinking. So radical were the ideas to Beverly, she left the office thinking, "this woman is off her rocker." When the traditional doctors gave her little hope for recovery, Beverly decided, at the advice of a spiritual counselor, to return to the nutritionist and follow her advice. Over the next year she strictly adhered to a macrobiotic diet, did positive affirmations, had daily ginger baths and massage, wore simple cotton clothing and watched funny movies to keep her spirits up. She also walked every day, even though she could only go about 800 feet at a time, and was exhausted by the effort.

Three months after changing her diet and lifestyle, Beverly's condition began to improve. "I can remember the turning point on August 17, 1984," she recalled. "That day my mouth, which was frozen almost completely shut, began to open a little, and I regained some movement in my lips. I knew that day I was going to beat this terrible disease."

Gradually throughout the next two years, Beverly's face began to unfreeze, her arms and legs lost their roughness, and her skin softened as her body slowly uncurled from its paralyzed state.

Prior to her illness Beverly had led a hectic lifestyle. She worked full time, took evening classes and was raising a teenage daughter alone. She described herself as "hot tempered and controlling." A perfectionist, she drove herself to the limit to do everything well. In addition, she was continually plagued with a fear of not doing or saying the right thing in front of people.

Growing up, Beverly's diet was the typical "meat and potatoes" with lots of sweets, especially chocolate. Being weight-conscious, she would strictly adhere to 1,200 calories a day, but the calories she counted often consisted of candy bars and junk food. Occasionally she would eat as much as a pound of chocolate in a day. She also had a five-year affair with Diet Pepsi, and drank a six pack almost every day for that time.

Beverly now shows few signs of the disease she fought over five years and that nearly took her life. The only remnants are seen in her fingers, which are curled up as if grasping a sheet of glass. She can do almost everything she did before getting sick, except completely open her fingers.

I asked Beverly what she thought helped her the most to survive this horrific illness and recover so remarkably. She said it was a combination of the macrobiotic diet, repeating mental affirmations that she would get well, and the help and support of her family and friends. In addition, she considers herself "an eternal optimist," and that while she prepared to die, she never surrendered to the thought. "I was determined to beat this," she said.

Beverly also attributes part of her healing to the medication she received and continues to take. While her doctor was never optimistic about her condition, he was amazed when she recovered so fully. He commented that he'd never seen anything like it before.

Beverly's plans include continuing with the macrobiotic diet indefinitely, as well as keeping up with the other positive changes she incorporated in her life over the past five years. She sees herself as a completely different person now than before getting sick. "I was inflexible, full of fears and very controlling. Now I'm more relaxed, peaceful, and happy most of the time. I love living every day."

With traces of the disease still in her fingers, Beverly continues to work on ways of improving her life and thinking. While currently taking a Dale Carnegie course to help alleviate her fears of public speaking and communicating with people, she believes that when she completely conquers these fears her fingers will be healed along with the rest of her body.

# Appendix: Classification of Yin and Yang

| Characteristic | YIN (▽)<br>Centrifugal Force | YANG (△)<br>Centripetal Force |
|---|---|---|
| Tendency | Expansion | Contraction |
| Function | Diffusion | Fusion |
| | Dispersion | Assimilation |
| | Separation | Gathering |
| | Decomposition | Organization |
| Movement | More inactive and slower | More active and faster |
| Vibration | Shorter wave and higher frequency | Longer wave and lower frequency |
| Direction | Ascent and vertical | Descent and horizontal |
| Position | More outward and peripheral | More inward and central |
| Weight | Lighter | Heavier |
| Temperature | Colder | Hotter |
| Light | Darker | Brighter |
| Humidity | More wet | More dry |
| Density | Thinner | Thicker |
| Size | Longer | Smaller |
| Shape | More expansive and fragile | More contractive and harder |
| Form | Longer | Shorter |
| Texture | Softer | Harder |
| Atomic particle | Electron | Proton |
| Elements | N, O, K, P, Ca, etc. | H, C, Na, As, Mg, etc. |
| Environment | Vibration . . . Air . . . Water . . . | Earth |
| Climatic effects | Tropical climate | Colder climate |
| Biology | More vegetable quality | More animal quality |
| Sex | Female | Male |
| Organ structure | More hollow and expansive | More compacted and condensed |
| Nerves | More peripheral, orthosympathetic | More central, parasympathetic |
| Attitude | More gentle, negative | More active, positive |
| Work | More psychological and mental | More physical and social |
| Dimension | Space | Time |

# Macrobiotic Resources——————

● **Macrobiotic Way of Life Seminar**

The *Macrobiotic Way of Life Seminar* is an introductory program offered by the Kushi Institute in Boston. It includes classes in macrobiotic cooking, home care, and kitchen setup, lectures on the philosophy of macrobiotics and the standard diet, and individual way of life guidance. It is presented monthly and includes introductory and intermediate level programs. Information on the *Macrobiotic Way of Life Seminar* is available from:

> The Kushi Institute
> 17 Station Street
> Brookline, Massachusetts 02147
> (617) 738–0045

● **Macrobiotic Residential Seminar**

The *Macrobiotic Residential Seminar* is an introductory program offered at the Kushi Foundation Berkshires Center in Becket, Massachusetts. It is a one week live-in program that includes hands-on training in macrobiotic cooking and home care, lectures on the philosophy and practice of macrobiotics, and meals prepared by a specially trained cooking staff. It is presented monthly and includes introductory and intermediate levels. Information on the *Macrobiotic Residential Seminar* is available from:

> Kushi Foundation Berkshires Center
> Box 7
> Becket, Massachusetts 01223
> (413) 623–5742

● **Kushi Institute Leadership Studies**

For those who wish to study further, the Kushi Institute in Boston offers instruction for individuals who wish to become trained and certified macrobiotic teachers. Similar leadership training programs are offered at Kushi Institute affiliates in London, Amsterdam, Antwerp, Florence, as well as in Portugal and Switzerland. Information on *Leadership Studies* is available from the Kushi Institute in Boston.

## • Other Programs

The Kushi Institute offers a variety of public programs including an annual Summer Conference in western Massachusetts, special weight-loss and natural beauty seminars, and intensive cooking and spiritual development training at the Berkshires Center. Information on these programs is available at either of the above addresses. Moreover, macrobiotic educational centers throughout the United States, Canada, and the world offer a variety of introductory and special programs. The Kushi Foundation publishes a *Worldwide Macrobiotic Directory* every year listing these centers and individuals. Please consult the *Directory* for the nearest macrobiotic center or qualified instructor.

## • Publications

Books and publications with information on macrobiotics are available from the Kushi Foundation, or at other macrobiotic centers, natural foodstores, and bookstores. Ongoing developments are reported in the Kushi Foundation's periodicals, including the *East West Journal*, a monthly magazine begun in 1971 and now with an international readership of 200,000. The *EWJ* features regular articles on the macrobiotic approach to health and nutrition, as well as related subjects. Moreover, Michio and Aveline Kushi have authored numerous books on macrobiotic philosophy, cooking, diet, and way of life. The following titles are especially recommended for further study:

## • Books by Michio Kushi

*Health and Diet*

---

1. *The Cancer-Prevention Diet* (with Alex Jack, St. Martin's Press, 1983)
2. *Diet for a Strong Heart* (with Alex Jack, St. Martin's Press, 1985)
3. *Natural Healing through Macrobiotics* (edited by Edward Esko and Marc Van Cauwenberghe, MD, Japan Publications, 1979)
4. *Macrobiotic Home Remedies* (edited by Marc Van Cauwenberghe, MD, Japan Publications, 1985)
5. *Macrobiotic Diet* (co-authored with Aveline Kushi; edited by Alex Jack, Japan Publications, 1985)
6. *Cancer and Heart Disease: The Macrobiotic Approach* (with various contributors; edited by Edward Esko, Japan Publications, 1982)
7. *Crime and Diet: The Macrobiotic Approach* (with various contributors; edited by Edward Esko, Japan Publications, 1987)

8. *AIDS: Cause and Solution—The Macrobiotic Approach to Natural Immunity* (co-authored with Martha C. Cottrell, MD, Japan Publications, 1988)

9. *Macrobiotic Health Education Series—Diabetes and Hypogylcemia; Allergies; Obesity, Weight Loss and Eating Disorders; Infertility and Reproductive Disorders; Stress and Hypertension* (with various editors, Japan Publications, 1985–88)

10. *How to See Your Health: the Book of Oriental Diagnosis* (Japan Publications, 1980)

11. *Your Face Never Lies* (Avery Publishing Group, 1983)

*Philosophy and Way of Life*

---

1. *One Peaceful World* (with Alex Jack, St. Martin's Press, 1986)

2. *The Book of Macrobiotics: The Universal Way of Health, Happiness, and Peace* (with Alex Jack, Japan Publications, revised edition, 1986)

3. *The Macrobiotic Way* (with Stephen Blauer, Avery Publishing Group, 1985)

4. *The Book of Do-In* (Japan Publications, 1979)

5. *Macrobiotic Palm Healing* (with Olivia Oredson Saunders, Japan Publications, 1988)

6. *On the Greater View* (Avery Publishing Group, 1986)

● **Books by Aveline Kushi**

*Cooking*

---

1. *Aveline Kushi's Complete Guide to Macrobiotic Cooking for Health, Harmony, and Peace* (with Alex Jack, Warner Books, 1985)

2. *Aveline Kushi's Introducing Macrobiotic Cooking* (with Wendy Esko, Japan Publications, 1987)

3. *The Changing Seasons Macrobiotic Cookbook* (with Wendy Esko, Avery Publishing Group, 1985)

4. *How to Cook with Miso* (Japan Publications, 1979)

5. *Macrobiotic Family Favorites* (with Wendy Esko, Japan Publications, 1987)

6. *The Macrobiotic Cancer Prevention Cookbook* (with Wendy Esko, Avery Publishing Group, 1988)

7. *Macrobiotic Food and Cooking Series—Diabetes and Hypogylcemia; Allergies; Obesity, Weight Loss and Eating Disorders; Infertility and Reproductive Disorders; Stress and Hypertension* (with various editors, Japan Publications, 1985–88)

1.   *Macrobiotic Pregnancy and Care of the Newborn* (with Michio Kushi; edited by Edward and Wendy Esko, Japan Publications, 1984)

2.   *Macrobiotic Child Care and Family Health* (with Michio Kushi; edited by Edward and Wendy Esko, Japan Publications, 1986)

3.   *Lessons of Night and Day* (Avery Publishing Group, 1985)

*Philosophy and Way of Life*

1.   *Aveline: The Life and Dream of the Woman Behind Macrobiotics Today* (with Alex Jack, Japan Publications, 1988)

In addition, macrobiotic publications by various authors are listed in the bibliography. These are also recommended for further study.

# Recommended Reading ────────────

## Books

Aihara, Cornellia. *The Dō of Cooking*. Chico, Calif.: George Ohsawa Macrobiotic Foundation, 1972.
────. *Macrobiotic Childcare*. Oroville, Calif.: George Ohsawa Macrobiotic Foundation, 1971.
────. *Macrobiotic Kitchen: Key to Good Health*. Tokyo & New York: Japan Publications, Inc., 1982.
Aihara, Herman. *Basic Macrobiotics*. Tokyo & New York: Japan Publications, Inc., 1985.
Benedict, Dirk. *Confessions of a Kamikaze Cowboy*. Van Nuys, Calif.: Newcastle, 1987.
Brown, Virginia, with Susan Stayman. *Macrobiotic Miracle: How a Vermont Family Overcame Cancer*. Tokyo & New York: Japan Publications, Inc., 1985.
*Dietary Goals for the United States*. Washington, D. C.: Select Committee on Nutrition and Human Needs, U.S. Senate, 1977.
*Diet, Nutrition, and Cancer*. Washington, D. C.: National Academy of Sciences, 1982.
Dufty, William. *Sugar Blues*. New York: Warner Books, 1975.
Esko, Wendy. *Aveline Kushi's Introducing Macrobiotic Cooking*. Tokyo & New York: Japan Publications, Inc., 1987.
Esko, Edward and Wendy. *Macrobiotic Cooking for Everyone*. Tokyo & New York: Japan Publications, Inc., 1980.
Esko, Edward, ed. *Doctors Look at Macrobiotics*. Tokyo & New York: Japan Publications, Inc., 1988.
Fukuoka, Masanobu. *The Natural Way of Farming*. Tokyo & New York: Japan Publications, Inc., 1985.
────. *The Road Back to Nature*. Tokyo & New York: Japan Publications, Inc., 1987.
────. *The One-Straw Revolution*. Emmaus, Pa.: Rodale Press, 1978.
*Healthy People: The Surgeon General's Report on Health Promotion and Disease Prevention*, Washington, D. C.: Government Printing Office, 1979.
Heidenry, Carolyn. *Making the Transition to a Macrobiotic Diet*. Wayne, N.J.: Avery Publishing Group, 1987.
Hippocrates. *Hippocratic Writings*. Edited by G. E. R. Lloyd. Trans-

128

lated by J. Chadwick and W. N. Mann. New York: Penguin Books, 1978.

*I Ching or Book of Changes*. Translated by Richard Wilhelm and Cary F. Baynes. Princeton: Bollingen Foundation, 1950.

Ineson, John. *The Way of Life: Macrobiotics and the Spirit of Christianity*. Tokyo & New York: Japan Publications, Inc., 1986.

Ishida, Eiwan. *Genmai: Brown Rice for Better Health*. Tokyo & New York: Japan Publications, Inc., 1988.

Jack, Gale with Alex Jack. *Promenade Home: Macrobiotics and Women's Health*. Tokyo & New York: Japan Publications, Inc., 1988.

Jacobs, Barbara and Leonard. *Cooking with Seitan: The Delicious Natural Food from Whole Grain*. Tokyo & New York: Japan Publications, Inc., 1986.

Jacobson, Michael. *The Changing American Diet*. Washington, D. C.: Center for Science in the Public Interest, 1978.

Kaibara, Ekiken. *Yojokun: Japanese Secrets of Good Health*. Tokyo: Tokuma Shoten, 1974.

Kidder, Ralph D. and Edward F. Kelly. *Choice for Survival: The Baby Boomer's Dilemma*. Tokyo & New York: Japan Pbulications, Inc., 1988.

Kohler, Jean and Mary Alice. *Healing Miracles from Macrobiotics*. West Nyack, N. Y.: Parker, 1979.

Kotzsch, Ronald. *Macrobiotics: Yesterday and Today*. Tokyo & New York: Japan Publications, Inc., 1985.

———. *Macrobiotics Beyond Food*. Tokyo & New York: Japan Publications, Inc., 1988.

Kushi, Aveline. *How to Cook with Miso*. Tokyo & New York: Japan Publications, Inc., 1978.

———. *Lessons of Night and Day*. Wayne, New Jersey: Avery Publishing Group, 1985.

———. *Macrobiotic Food and Cooking Series: Diabetes and Hypoglycemia; Allergies*. Tokyo & New York: Japan Publications, Inc., 1985.

———. *Macrobiotic Food and Cooking Series: Obesity, Weight Loss, and Eating Disorders; Infertility and Reproductive Disorders*. Tokyo & New York: Japan Publications, Inc., 1987.

Kushi, Aveline, with Alex Jack. *Aveline Kushi's Complete Guide to Macrobiotic Cooking*. New York: Warner Books, 1985.

———. *Aveline: The Life and Dream of the Woman Behind Macrobiotics Today*. Tokyo & New York: Japan Publications, Inc., 1988.

Kushi, Aveline and Michio. *Macrobiotic Pregnancy and Care of the Newborn*. Edited by Edward and Wendy Esko. Tokyo & New York: Japan Publications, Inc., 1984.

129

———. *Macrobiotic Child Care and Family Health.* Tokyo & New York: Japan Publications, Inc., 1986.

Kushi, Aveline, and Wendy Esko. *Macrobiotic Family Favorites.* Tokyo & New York: Japan Publications, Inc., 1987.

Kushi, Aveline, and Wendy Esko. *The Changing Seasons Macrobiotic Cookbook.* Wayne, N. J.: Avery Publishing Group, 1983.

———. *The Macrobiotic Cancer Prevention Cookbook.* Wayne, New Jersey: Avery Publishing Group, 1986.

Kushi, Michio. *The Book of Dō-In: Exercise for Physical and Spiritual Development.* Tokyo & New York: Japan Publications, Inc., 1979.

———. *The Book of Macrobiotics: The Universal Way of Health, Happiness and Peace.* Tokyo & New York: Japan Publications, Inc., 1986 (Rev. ed.).

———. *Cancer and Heart Disease: The Macrobiotic Approach to Degenerative Disorders.* Tokyo & New York: Japan Publications, Inc., 1986 (Rev. ed.).

———. *Crime and Diet: The Macrobiotic Approach.* Tokyo & New York: Japan Publications, Inc., 1987.

———. *The Era of Humanity.* Brookline, Mass.: East West Journal, 1980.

———. *How to See Your Health: The Book of Oriental Diagnosis.* Tokyo & New York: Japan Publications, Inc., 1980.

———. *Macrobiotic Health Education Series: Diabetes and Hypoglycemia; Allergies.* Tokyo & New York: Japan Publications, Inc., 1985.

———. *Macrobiotic Health Education Series: Obesity, Weight Loss, and Eating Disorders; Infertility and Reproductive Disorders.* Tokyo & New York: Japan Publications, Inc., 1987.

———. *Natural Healing through Macrobiotics.* Tokyo & New York: Japan Publications, Inc., 1978.

———. *On the Greater View: Collected Thoughts on Macrobiotics and Humanity.* Wayne, New Jersey: Avery Publishing Group, 1985.

———. *Your Face Never Lies.* Wayne, N. J.: Avery Publishing Group, 1983.

Kushi, Michio, and Alex Jack. *The Cancer-Prevention Diet.* New York: St. Martin's Press, 1983.

———. *Diet for a Strong Heart.* New York: St. Martin's Press, 1984.

Kushi, Michio, with Alex Jack. *One Peaceful World.* New York: St. Martin's Press, 1987.

Kushi, Michio and Aveline, with Alex Jack. *The Macrobiotic Diet.* Tokyo & New York: Japan Publications, Inc., 1985.

Kushi, Michio and Martha C. Cottrell. *AIDS: Cause and Solution— The Macrobiotic Approach to Natural Immunity.* Tokyo & New York:

Japan Publications, Inc., 1988.

Kushi, Michio, and the East West Foundation. *The Macrobiotic Approach to Cancer*. Wayne, N. J.: Avery Publishing Group, 1982.

Kushi, Michio, with Stephen Blauer. *The Macrobiotic Way*. Wayne, New Jersey: Avery Publishing Group, 1985.

Kushi, Michio with Olivia Oredson. *Macrobiotic Palm Healing: Energy at Your Finger-tips*. Tokyo & New York: Japan Publications, Inc., 1988.

Levin, Cecile Tovah. *Cooking for Regeneration: Macrobiotic Relief from Cancer, AIDS, and Degenerative Disease*. Tokyo & New York: Japan Publications, Inc., 1988.

Mendelsohn, Robert S., M.D. *Confessions of a Medical Heretic*. Chicago: Contemporary Books, 1979.

———. *Male Practice*. Chicago: Contemporary Books, 1980.

Nussbaum, Elaine. *Recovery: From Cancer to Health through Macrobiotics*. Tokyo & New York: Japan Publications, Inc., 1986.

*Nutrition and Mental Health*. Washington, D. C.: Select Committee on Nutrition and Human Needs, U.S. Senate, 1977, 1980.

Ohsawa, George, *Cancer and the Philosophy of the Far East*. Oroville, Calif.: George Ohsawa Macrobiotic Foundation, 1971 edition.

———. *You Are All Sanpaku*. Edited by William Dufty, New York: University Books, 1965.

———. *Zen Macrobiotics*. Los Angeles: Ohsawa Foundation, 1965.

Ohsawa, Lima. *Macrobiotic Cuisine*. Tokyo & New York: Japan Publications, Inc., 1984.

Polatin, Betsy. *Macrobiotics in Motion: Yin and Yang in Moving Spirals*. Tokyo & New York: Japan Publications, Inc., 1987.

Price, Western, A., D.D.S. *Nutrition and Physical Degeneration*. Santa Monica, Calif.: Price-Pottenger Nutritional Foundation, 1945.

Sattilaro, Anthony, M.D., with Tom Monte. *Recalled by Life: The Story of My Recovery from Cancer*. Boston: Houghton-Mifflin, 1982.

Schauss, Alexander. *Diet, Crime, and Delinquency*. Berkeley, Calif.: Parker House, 1980.

Scott, Neil E., with Jean Farmer. *Eating with Angels*. Tokyo & New York: Japan Publications, Inc., 1986.

Sergel, David. *The Macrobiotic Way of Zen Shiatsu*. Tokyo & New York: Japan Publications, Inc., 1988.

Tara, William. *A Challenge to Medicine*. Tokyo & New York: Japan Publications, Inc., 1988.

———. *Macrobiotics and Human Behavior*. Tokyo & New York: Japan Publications, Inc., 1985.

Wood, Rebecca. *Quinoa the Supergrain: Ancient Food for Today*. Tokyo & New York: Japan Publications, Inc., 1988.

Yamamoto, Shizuko. *Barefoot Shiatsu*. Tokyo & New York: Japan Publications, Inc., 1979.

*The Yellow Emperor's Classic of Internal Medicine*. Translated by Ilza Veith, Berkeley: University of California Press, 1949.

## Periodicals

*East West Journal*. Brookline, Mass.

*Macromuse*. Washington, D. C.

*Nutrition Action*. Washington, D. C.

"The People's Doctor" by Robert S. Mendelsohn, M.D. and Marian Tompson, Evanston, Ill.

# Index